Sexuality and Addiction

Making Connections,
Enhancing Recovery

Raven L. James

Foreword by Douglas Braun-Harvey

Sabrena,
well, here we are again — finally! reconnecting after all these years! The universe has plans for us as we prepare to rule the world and create some awesome new realities :) we are aligned once more. I look forward to being back would ✦ sexual health with you. Love, Raven

PRAEGER

AN IMPRINT OF ABC-CLIO, LLC
Santa Barbara, California • Denver, Colorado • Oxford, England

Library of Congress Cataloging-in-Publication Data

James, Raven L.
   Sexuality and addiction : making connections, enhancing recovery / Raven L. James ; foreword by Douglas Braun-Harvey.
      p. ; cm.
   Includes bibliographical references and index.
   ISBN 978–0–313–39635–9 (hardback : alk. paper) — ISBN 978–0–313–39636–6 (e-ISBN)
   I. Title.
   [DNLM: 1. Substance-Related Disorders—therapy. 2. Sexual Behavior. 3. Sexuality.
4. Substance-Related Disorders—complications. WM 270]

616.85′8—dc23   2012005644

ISBN: 978–0–313–39635–9
EISBN: 978–0–313–39636–6

16 15 14 13 12   1 2 3 4 5

This book is also available on the World Wide Web as an eBook.
Visit www.abc-clio.com for details.

Praeger
An Imprint of ABC-CLIO, LLC

ABC-CLIO, LLC
130 Cremona Drive, P.O. Box 1911
Santa Barbara, California 93116-1911

This book is printed on acid-free paper (∞)

Manufactured in the United States of America

Portions of this book were adapted from:
James, Raven. "Strategies for Incorporating Women-Specific Sexuality Education into Addiction Treatment Models." *American Journal of Sexuality Education* 2(3), 3–25, 2007.

To Ken, my greatest love in my life,
thank you for teaching me how to believe in love again.
Like the moon and the stars in the sky,
always and forever . . .

Contents

Foreword

I keep finding sexual health angels.

In 2001, I was asked to help a residential drug and alcohol treatment program in San Diego, California, stop kicking their clients out of treatment, not for getting high but for having sex. Cheryl Houk, then executive director of Stepping Stone, said, "Too many of our residents are relapsing because of their sexual behavior." She wanted to find a way to address sexual behavior during and after treatment to "stop the dying." "We can do better."

It did not take long to find that there indeed were a significant number of Stepping Stone clients whose treatment failure was inextricably linked with their sexual behavior. In 2002, I traveled the country asking treatment providers how they addressed sexual-linked relapse. They would ask me if I meant treating sexual addiction. Or they would correct me: "You mean survivors of sexual abuse." Many times the subject moved immediately to the topic of men and women getting in relationships with other clients in treatment. I began to see a predictable pattern among drug and alcohol treatment programs and counselors. Sexuality could be talked about as a problem (addiction, abuse, relationships) but not as an ally for helping women and men recover. I also became increasingly worried that something was wrong. It was not just Stepping Stone that needed to do better.

Over the next five years, I collaborated with Stepping Stone to pioneer the nation's first sex/drug-linked relapse prevention program. Our goal was to increase client retention as well as provide proactive sexual health recovery tools for men and women with sex/drug-linked patterns of addiction. We did not do this alone. Many sexual health-in-recovery allies came forward. The California Endowment funded a three-year study. National addiction treatment conferences and sexual health conferences welcomed me to inform them of this new idea of sexual health in recovery as a means for improving treatment and decreasing risk of sex-linked relapse. National leaders in sexuality and drug and alcohol treatment endorsed the need to end the avoidance of sexuality within drug and alcohol treatment. Most heartening was to find individual drug and alcohol treatment counselors who were already quietly discussing sex with their clients. The problem was they were not counseling clients on sex related to recovery because of a program policy or training or because of specific direction from their supervisor. They were like Cheryl. They saw the problem—the terrible risk for sexuality-related treatment failure—and rather than support the status quo, they decided to address the issue. I think they were sick of watching people relapse in part because their treatment and recovery program was avoiding addressing a central aspect of many clients' addiction: sex/drug-linked patterns of addiction.

I started calling these women and men drug and alcohol treatment sexual health angels. They seemed like angels because they would just appear from among the attendees at my workshops, send an email after I spoke at a conference, or just write me to introduce them and tell me of their work. I would also advise them that if they wanted real change in how sex is addressed in addiction treatment, they could not do it alone. The sexual health angels in drug and alcohol treatment cannot single-handedly do the work of change.

This is how I came to meet Raven James. Both members of the Society for the Scientific Study of Sexuality, Raven sought me out as a result of our common interest in principles of sexual health improving drug and alcohol treatment. It was clear that Raven was more than an individual who identified the need for sexual health relapse prevention and surreptitiously talking with her clients about sex. Raven had much more in mind. She wanted things to change. As a trained sex researcher and professor at Governors State University, I had now met an ally in a position to apply her vision of sexual health in recovery. It was in this moment that I began to sense what the sexual health in recovery angels may have felt when greeting me. I felt relieved, optimistic, and eager to talk and discuss her perspectives on sexual health–based sex/drug-linked relapse prevention. With *Sexuality and Addiction: Making Connections, Enhancing Recovery*, Raven makes a much-needed addition to the repertoire of early books on this topic. This book combines her personal process with in-depth sexual health science to invite the reader to reflect on his or her own process of working with the sexual issues of clients in drug and alcohol treatment.

Her book is the beginning of many necessary new and vibrant voices and perspectives on integrating sexual health in drug and alcohol treatment not only to improve treatment but to save lives as well. I am grateful for Raven adding her voice for the men and women in drug and alcohol treatment waiting to get their sexual health angel wings.

Douglas Braun-Harvey, MA, MFT, CGP, CST
San Diego, California

Preface

Log on to the Internet and conduct a search on sex and addiction or on sexuality and addiction. Page upon page of sex addiction, compulsive sexual behaviors, cybersex, and the like are the majority of hits. But it's not what you're looking for. You're a drug and alcohol counselor searching for information on sexuality issues to help your clients in treatment. Not that this entry yields a better result; much of it is still related to sex addiction. You have recognized that many individuals you work with not only are relapsing because of sexuality issues but have confided in you that their drug use is inextricably connected to their substance use, yet the dearth of existing resources has you exacerbated.

The frustration over the paucity of sexual health research in the literature on sexuality education for people in addictions treatment is part of what led me to write this book.

MY BACKGROUND IN SEXUALITY AND ADDICTION

I have worked in the field of addictions and sexual health since 1994 and also have a PhD in human sexuality. I worked with substance-abusing clients at an AIDS organization in the 1990s, providing HIV and sexuality education to drug and alcohol clients and staff throughout New York State. Through my community-based work, I literally served thousands of people. The most challenging of all the people I worked with were the providers. Sure, my clients challenged me at times, but their issues were easier for me to resolve because they responded more readily to the information and techniques I used with them. The providers were another story. Often they squirmed and balked about incorporating sexuality-related issues into treatment programming. Many counselors were often relieved to be able to discuss sex, eager to learn, and grateful for the assistance I provided, yet administratively I was often prevented from doing more in-depth exploration of sexual topics. Some of the reasons were based out of fear, fear that people would relapse if they talked too early in treatment about sexuality issues. The truth of the matter is that the relapse rate for people in recovery from drug and alcohol use is already high; almost 40 to 60 percent of people with substance abuse problems will experience a relapse as part of the recovery process (National Institute for Drug Abuse, 2011). And while relapse is part of the change process, a great deal of it stems from unaddressed sexuality issues. So by not talking about sex with clients, we do potential harm to them and contribute to the relapse process.

Part of my work for providers included teaching HIV-related updates and topics and sexuality-related topics. What I mean in this case by sexuality-related topics included sexuality transmitted infections and HIV information, sexual identity, domestic violence, safer sex, and sexual risk related to counseling issues in drug and alcohol treatment. These included epidemiology, behavior change theory, and techniques to assist counselors in helping their clients acknowledge sexual risk, seek testing, and reduce or eliminate harmful sexual and drug using practices that could lead to HIV or sexuality transmitted infections. For some reason, many of the professionals seemed more uncomfortable with discussing sexual matters than their clients. I hypothesized that this had to do with the lack of comfort with and knowledge of sexual issues, in part, as well as from unresolved issues of their own sexual pasts. Considering the fact that many drug and alcohol counselors are also in recovery themselves, they may have had similar sexuality-related experiences that were unaddressed and now threatened to undermine their confidence in treating clients.

Another component of my work consisted of providing HIV overviews and sexuality-related topics to clients of drug and alcohol agencies. In New York State, the Office of Alcohol and Substance Abuse Services (OASAS) mandates that all clients who go through drug and alcohol treatment receive HIV information. This is due to the fact that New York State has the highest rate of HIV/AIDS in the country, and there are many links to substance abuse and HIV risk (Centers for Disease Control and Prevention, 2009). AIDS service providers in New York State have OASAS-funded positions that do much of this work. So, if a person were to go through treatment 10 times, they would receive the standard HIV overview 10 times. This was the extent of sexuality education for clients in the treatment process—not very comprehensive if you ask me. Sexuality is linked to drug use in very intimate ways; therefore, it stands to reason that we must delve deeper to effectively help folks recover. I am here to assist you on this journey.

Beyond the HIV overview, some of my more meaningful client work included the development of sexuality-related trainings for clients. A couple of agencies recognized the sexuality-related relapse in their clients and welcomed the opportunity for a sexuality-based psychoeducational program. I developed and piloted a sexuality program for women in treatment that incorporated a holistic view of sexual health. You see, sexuality is a complex entity. It consists of many parts that make us who we are as sexual beings, including intimacy, sexual identity, sexual health and reproduction, sensuality, and sexualization. If you don't know what all these components entail, that is exactly my point. The information contained in these pages will provide a comprehensive overview of how sexuality is intimately linked to addiction and provide the impetus to form new frameworks of understanding sexual health in recovery.

Acknowledgments

No book is ever written in a vacuum. There are many individuals who contributed to the process of this work, both direct and indirectly. First and foremost are the clients who willingly shared their lived experiences with me in the spirit of sexual health in recovery. Without your stories, the voices of those we serve would be missing. Next, thank you to all the people at Praeger/ABC-CLIO who made this work a reality. To a few of my many mentors and colleagues in the field of sexual health—Konnie McCaffree, PhD; Bill Stayton, ThD; Lori Simons, PhD; and especially Douglas Braun-Harvey—for inspiring me to take my passion for sexual health further into the field of addiction. Special thanks to Jasmine Williams for spending hours of your time compiling resources (when you should have been working on your homework). Todd Burd, thank you for your sense of humor and willingness to share some of your life and work with body image across the life span. Margaret Brady and Cindy Olczyk, your help with proofreading and thoughtful comments helped me stay focused. Jeanine Klomes and Jessica Hudak, I gratefully thank you for helping take care of those 12 horses in my barn so I could get through the home stretch. Last, but not least, I thank my mom, who continually provides support and meaning to my life. To all of you who have contributed to my professional development and helped me finish this project, I am grateful.

Introduction

We live in a society that is sexually ignorant, sexually traumatized, and sexually secretive. The Puritans were responsible, in part, for setting a prudent sexual climate, and although sexual images bombard us today in the media, we typically don't talk to our kids about how to understand and process this information. We *don't know how*, or we are *embarrassed*. Nor will we collectively allow comprehensive sexuality education to be a part of the K–12 school curriculum. We are *afraid* to talk to youth about sex because we think that they will go out and have sex, lots of it, and that this will harm them. Nothing could be further from the truth.

The truth of the matter is that sex is normal and natural and beautiful. Sex is not about engaging in indiscriminate sexual acts, although this is a form of sexual expression. Sex is not about fear or hate or perversion. But sex gets a bad rap. It causes all these negative consequences, AIDS syphilis, teenage pregnancy, and rape, right? Wrong again. What actually causes the problems, in part, revolves around the fact that *we don't know what sex is*, we are afraid of it, and we *haven't learned enough to be able to have enough comfort* around the subject to *communicate*.

If we could just learn how to talk about sex, really talk about it, life would be a whole lot less complicated. People might understand what unhealthy relationships looked like and feel good enough about themselves that they could avoid domestic violence, unwanted pregnancies, and disease. They might know how to negotiate the use of birth control and safer sex methods and feel good enough about themselves to use them or masturbate or abstain. They might know the difference between love and lust or mistaking sex for love and having sex to get attention to feel loved. They might not feel so ashamed of their sexual selves to have to turn to alcohol or drugs in order not to feel, to numb the pain of love gone badly, or to drink to reduce their inhibitions in order to be sexual.

But how would counselors have enough of this knowledge when the lack of information is coupled with elements such as poverty, violence, racism, homophobia, loss, co-occurring disorders, life transitions, sexual prejudice, and such? Life is complicated enough without knowing how to navigate relationships and sex. So, some people get all screwed up and start a pattern of substance abuse in order to help them cope. Some of them end up in jail, institutions, or treatment, or, worse, they die. And once they are caught up in systems, treatment can be complicated. We expect a lot when we ask our clients to focus on their substance abuse and don't address some of the key issues that kept them using, or can trigger their relapses—namely, issues related to sex.

It's akin to telling diabetics to use their insulin but without a needle. If we don't have a basic understanding of what sexuality is, how can we help out clients navigate a successful recovery? Many of their substance abuse issues are so intertwined with sexuality that we can't talk about one without addressing the other. And if we do not talk about sexuality, we do harm by not presenting the entire picture.

Typically, areas of sexuality not discussed in treatment include those pertaining to sensuality, intimacy, sexual identity, and sexualization. These areas, for many, are the areas that cause them shame, confusion, trauma, low self-esteem, poor body image, eating disorders, self-hatred, homophobia, sexual dysfunction, poor communication skills, failed relationships, and more. Interrupting the internal process and negative self-dialogue are the areas that need to be addressed for people in treatment programs in order for them to successfully recover and help prevent relapse. Many relapse triggers for substance users include latent, unresolved sexual issues. Addressing sexuality in treatment programs can provide a baseline for new understanding and assist counselors in setting up vital follow-up treatment plans that include awareness and understanding of sexuality issues that may need further therapy, support, and intervention. This book is written to provide this understanding so that counselors may make the sexuality and addiction links in a positive manner.

WHO CAN BENEFIT FROM READING THIS BOOK?

The information presented in this book is geared primarily for counselors or other health professionals working with substance users who are searching for sexuality information related to their clients. Although clinicians may have a solid foundation in supporting clients in the treatment process, little to no training in sexual health is offered in addiction counseling programs (both at the college level and through state-funded training). Historically, sex has not been broached in treatment programs from a positive model. Often, sex is viewed negatively, swept under the rug, and ignored in both treatment programs and self-help groups. The main goal of this book is to provide substance abuse counselors with a broad grounding in sexuality issues and clear identification of sexual links to addiction and the recovery process. It is my goal for you as a professional counselor to develop comfort and skill in fostering a positive sexually healthy environment for clients to recover in within your agency. I also provide some background and history of how certain sexual topics have shaped our attitudes in the hope that this can help you to identify personal bias and not allow it to interfere with your client work.

Although the book is written with the drug and alcohol professional in mind, family members and loved ones will also find some useful information within the chapters that can help you understand the connections between sexuality and addictive behaviors, discover ways to support and approach your loved one with compassion, and provide hope for positive sexual health outcomes. If you are a recovery coach or someone who provides ancillary support, this book will provide a baseline knowledge level and guide you toward further training and resources for professional development. It is not intended to replace professional training in facilitating sexual health groups. Finally, if you are a recovering person or someone struggling with substance misuse, the information presented here can assist you in developing an understanding of how sexuality may have impacted your use of alcohol and other drugs or vice versa. Internalizing this knowledge can help you develop healthier intimate relationships, identify possible relapse triggers, and offer suggestions for reversing sexually shaming messages.

A ROAD MAP

The goal of this book is to provide an in-depth, easy-to-understand road map of what sexuality entails and how it relates to the addiction recovery process. It explains why we need to talk about it and how we can do that. It also gives many examples of how trained counselors can incorporate discussions, activities, and issues into existing groups and suggests ideas for stand-alone groups that address certain topics, such as gender-specific or lesbian, gay, bisexual, and transgender issues. Several tools are also presented that can assist counselors to assess and serve clients in the treatment setting. Within this framework, keep in mind that as a counselor you will need to develop comfort and skills in addition to knowledge of sexuality issues in order to effectively implement some of the activities into the treatment setting.

STRUCTURE

Each chapter in this book provides a general introduction to the selected topic, discusses connections to substance use and relapse through the lived narratives of clients, and provides detailed scientific evidence to connect sexuality and addiction and then suggests ways for counselors to enhance the recovery process of clients (or themselves if they are recovering). Suggestions for working with groups through counselor tips, tools, and related sexuality lessons are included within the specific framework of each topic, usually near each chapter's conclusion. The chapter format varies from chapter to chapter in terms of how the various tips, tools, and lessons are interwoven with the sexuality material.

OVERVIEW

Chapter 1 introduces a sexual health model from which the topics of the book will be based and discusses the concept of sexual self-esteem and how it can be utilized to measure sexual health improvements and as a brief assessment tool.

Chapter 2 incorporates material on definitions, clarifies confusing terminology, and introduces activities that can be used to desensitize folks to sexual language; it is the cornerstone of sexual health. Methods for discussing one's own sexual values, preferences, attractions, history, and behavior are introduced. Sexual communication is a necessary skill for sexual health and must be learned and practiced in order to be effective with potential sexual partners. Ideas for activities are included that practitioners can use in groups to encourage the use of positive communication with sexual behaviors.

Chapter 3 discusses the impact of culture and sexual identity and describes the complexities of human difference with regard to defining ourselves as sexual beings. Terminology related to sexual orientation, gender identity, and gender is introduced. Several assessment tools are presented for use with sexual identity development and coming-out issues.

Chapter 4 covers basic knowledge around sexual anatomy, reproductive functioning, and sexual response in relation to substance use and addiction problems. Knowledge on how to enable clients to discuss sexual issues with more comfort and to identify feelings and attitudes associated with relapse triggers is also introduced.

Chapter 5 includes a section on safer sex and sexual health self-care. Its broad perspective incorporates knowledge about sexual self-care related to sexually transmitted infections/HIV, birth control, and reproductive issues to lower the risk of sexual health risks. The meanings of safer sex and unsafe sexual practices are explored with regard to gender, race, and sexual orientation. Methods to explore this individually or in groups is covered.

Chapter 6 includes information on how to talk about traumatic sexual experiences, including abuse, sexual harassment, compulsive sexual behavior, and discrimination. These experiences can increase the risk and vulnerability for misusing substances as well as increase the risk for relapse if not addressed in treatment. Methods for improving sexual functioning and fostering a decreased need for the use of substances to overcome inhibitions are explained.

Chapter 7 discusses body image across the life span, which is an important aspect of sexual health and can be directly related to unhealthy practices through behaviors such as binging and purging, using amphetamines to suppress appetite, and compulsive exercise. These aspects of body image are discussed with regard to relapse triggers and enhancing personal body esteem through the use of experiential activities that can be modified for gender and sexual orientation issues in treatment.

Chapter 8 incorporates the concept of fantasy and masturbation in relation to sexual health and safer sex. Fantasy is a normal part of sexuality and, when used appropriately, can enhance a partnership between individuals. We live in a culture that views masturbation as a moral deficiency, and examining these views with regard to the ensuing shame that is associated with the behavior can increase the likelihood of fostering positive sexual self-esteem. Individuals also can learn about their own sexual responses through safe exploration of their own bodies and reduce the risk of disease. Recommended films and activities are included.

Chapter 9 introduces a positive sexual self-concept, something that is typically absent from an addicted individual's life. Sexuality is discussed and explored through the use of skill-building activities that foster communication about sexual pleasure and boundary setting. Rather than viewing sexuality from a deficit, disease concept, sexual health is explored in terms of positive, healthy self-regard.

Chapter 10 is about how to be intimate in a relationship. Society upholds the value that intimacy is about sex when, in fact, intimacy is about the ability to be close to another human being and have that close-ness returned. This includes a variety of relationships, nonsexual as well as sexual. Many substance-abusing persons have learned unhealthy sexual practices that mimic intimacy through sexual behavior and can benefit from learning new perspectives to view intimacy in a broader context. This chapter includes ideas for activities that foster the development and knowledge of how to achieve these views.

Chapter 11 talks about the connection that individuals have in relation to their spirituality, which, in the case of substance abusers, is often about feeling morally deficient. Religion, which is the formal practice under which spirituality is "housed," can bring about feelings of shame and eth-ical concerns. Reclaiming one's spirituality with regard to sexuality and religion can be empowering for someone who has internalized shaming sexual messages.

Chapter 12 is a brief reflection of the journey around the wheel of sexual health and the lessons we have learned along the way as well as my hopes for revolutionizing the way we work with clients in treatment settings.

This book weaves my professional processes with scientific sexuality research and a sexuality education framework. I move from the experiential to the technical as relevant material is presented. Feel free to borrow any or all of these activities and ideas for use in your clinical settings; just do your clients a favor and talk about sex. They will thank you, and so will I.

ONE

Models of Sexual Health and Sexual Self-Esteem

Now I've gotten you here; let's get down to it. Besides all the nuts and bolts of sex, I want to give you some basic understanding of what it's all about. I remember when I first learned about sex. No, not the first time I "did it" but the first time I really got the real deal. It was 1999, and it changed my world. I was working for an AIDS organization in upstate New York and got to go to Sex Camp. In actuality, it was a Sexuality Attitude Reassessment (SAR), but Sex Camp is what it was dubbed by those who had gone before me.

SEX CAMP

At Sex Camp, you learn everything you ever wanted to know about sex. From birth to death, we are sexual beings. Even in utero, girls' vaginas lubricate and boys have erections. And 90-year-old people can still have sexual relations and be intimate with their partners. Sure, not everyone is sexual with partners that late in life, but if people are fortunate enough to be sexual, they are. There were such topics as child sexual development, puberty, masturbation, sexual identity, pornography, sexual pleasure, safer sex, family constellations, relationships, fertility, and more. The sky was the limit. We watched movies, did small- and large-group work, and processed, experienced, and learned about ourselves. We learned about our values, beliefs, and attitudes toward sexuality. Our buttons were pushed, and we reevaluated what we knew, what we thought we knew, and information we never knew. It was life altering for me, and

I felt cheated growing up never having had such a broad knowledge base of what sexuality was actually all about. I'm not sure many of us are lucky enough to have been raised with such comprehensive learning.

SEXUAL BEINGNESS

One of my favorite teaching tools I have encountered for introductory sexuality group work is called Sexual Beingness. I first encountered this tool from a colleague who was introduced to it at Sex Camp, and we adapted it to develop a sexuality group for women in treatment. Sexual Beingness was derived from a similar model called the Circles of Sexuality (Advocates for Youth, 2011). The illustration in Figure 1.1 depicts its content adapted for this book.

Each circle represents a different aspect of sexuality; each bolded phrase represents a different chapter in this book. When you first viewed the constellation, what is one thing that you noticed about the circles? They are all connected. I like to reference Native American teachings when I introduce the circles of sexuality. In many indigenous cultures, the circle is representative of life's never-ending cycle (birth, death, and rebirth). Circles have been represented by medicine wheels or mandalas in Native American teachings. The medicine wheel is a symbol of symmetry and balance and represents the many cycles of life. Each circle or spoke placement in the wheel focuses on a different aspect of living and has been defined by some as the four directions, although other definitions exist. The four directions can also represent the emotional, spiritual, mental, and physical aspects of ourselves as human beings. When one of the areas is impacted, it affects all the other areas on the wheel. This concept is one that I learned about through my work in addictions recovery: treat the whole person, not just the parts. It's the same thing with sexuality: if a person is having difficulty in one of the circles, that ripple effect occurs in the others; all are connected. For many of our clients, various spokes of their sexuality wheel have been harmed, and this affects their lives in many ways. We can use the circles and their attributes to teach about sexuality from a holistic perspective, thus promoting healing and harmony.

The Blue-Light Special

Another question for you: which circle is the most familiar? Sexual health and reproduction. We sexologists fondly refer to this circle as the "blue-light special." Attention, K-Mart shoppers, we are having a special on vibrators, lube, and condoms in the health and beauty aisle. That's

Figure 1.1   Adapted from Life Planning Education. Advocates for Youth, Washington, DC, www.advocatesforyouth.org. Circles of Sexuality created by Dennis M. Dailey, Professor Emeritus, University of Kansas, based on the initial work of Harvey Gochros.

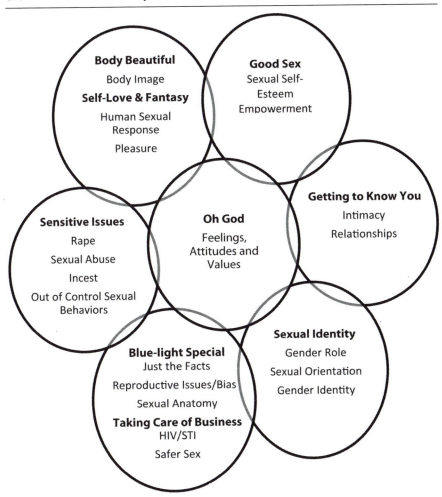

the sexual health and beauty aisle to you return shoppers. If we learned anything growing up about sex, this was the area we learned about. I say *if* because, sadly, many schools did not or do not offer sex education at all, and some receive and are bound by federal funding that can mandate an abstinence-only curriculum. Now *that* will *not* help our sexually active youth make sound decisions around safer sex. I think that providing abstinence education is important but comprises only one small cog in the wheel. We need to consider the bigger picture where sexuality is concerned.

SOURCES OF SEXUAL LEARNING

Because honestly folks, how many of you learned about sex from your parents while you were growing up? C'mon, show of hands here. Did anyone learn about sex from the church? Oh, more hands are raised now. What is that? You learned negative things? How about your friends? Ah, more hands are raising now. Oh no, you got chlamydia from your friends? Now that sounds very likely. And with today's friends with benefits, youth may get more than they bargained for: human papillomavirus, herpes, and HIV—not exactly the bacterial craze anymore. At least antibiotics could cure those. Viruses are for life.

Seriously, when we consider the source of our learning, the depth of the information, and the spirit in which the information was given, the likelihood that it was healthy and sex positive seems low. I like to pose these questions because our clients learned about sex in similar ways to ourselves or worse. A client had shared with me about coming home with crabs as a teenager and having to tell her mother because she had no idea how to get rid of the critters. The mother told the young girl that she was nasty, dirty, and disgusting. Those messages stayed with her psyche for a long time and shaped her sexual self-esteem. It is not unusual for parents to react negatively to their adolescents' sexual experiences with punitive, shameful responses; it is more of the norm. Living in a culture that does not embrace adolescent sexuality as part of development does not foster communication between teens and their parents, and contributes to secrecy and internalized messages of guilt and shame.

I remember being assigned a paper to write in one of my graduate classes about why we were pursuing a degree in human sexuality and to muse about how others might react to that knowledge. For example, would they be suspect of us somehow and make judgments and assumptions about who we are as people? The truth of the matter is that people do get stereotyped, labeled, and even branded for doing this kind of work. We are out on a limb, sometimes viewed by conservatives as potential child molesters, perverts, sickos, and queers. The point of the exercise was not to scare us away but to have us honestly examine our motives, become more aware of how society may react, and prepare us for the long haul. I already felt prepared to some degree, based on my work in HIV and substance abuse. People can be cruel, so I cannot imagine how degraded one of my gay, African American, HIV-positive, drug-using clients must have felt when ostracized and shunned by society, his own family, and community for aspects of his identity.

Feelings, Values, and Attitudes

You might be wondering how this all relates to sex. If you check out the glue that holds the circles together, "Oh God," it also contains feelings, values, and attitudes. How can we talk about sex and sexuality if we don't discuss our feelings, values, and attitudes? Just the facts, ma'am—the woman's ovary releases the egg, and when the sperm reach that egg, it can become fertilized, resulting in a woman's pregnancy. Now, that is compelling and factual. Leave the rest of life and circumstance out of that conversation, and youth will surely know how to negotiate relationships and engage in safer, healthy sexual practices. I would dare to say most schools aren't discussing ectopic pregnancies, spontaneous abortions, and emergency contraception, let alone abortion. We don't want to open the floodgates to hell. Do we think by not talking about it that it won't happen? Kids won't have sex, get pregnant, and have babies or abortions?

What do we tell youth? Do we tell them that sex is bad, dirty, and not legal until they are 18 or that they should wait until marriage to have sex? What happens to the lesbian and gay youth who can't get married in most states; should they just not be allowed to be sexual at all? We tell youth plenty through our words and actions. They learn how to treat others based on what they see adults do and what comes out of their mouths. So, when Dad tells fag jokes at the dinner table (or worse) and everyone laughs, we teach a strong lesson. Youth form their values and beliefs, in part, from what they see and hear going on around them and typically behave based on the norms of their peer groups. The feelings and attitudes formed in childhood and adolescence shape the direction youth will take in life. We have such rich opportunities to talk to our kids about sex, values, feelings, and attitudes but often choose not to because of our own embarrassment, ignorance, or internal shame.

Without the words or the ability to communicate with adults, youth can be seduced down a path of shame and fear, like the kid who comes home with crabs, is grounded by her mother, and continues to use drugs to cover up the feelings of shame. For youth who have multiple risk factors, the onset of sexual experience often coincides with a substance, be it alcohol or some other drug. Risk factors commonly include low self-esteem, a parent who uses drugs, divorce, trauma, abuse, environment, and so on. Multiple risk, multiple trauma, and co-occurring disorders (mental health issues) can lead to long-term problematic substance use and abuse. We, as counselors, family members, and recovery support persons, need to understand the links between sexuality issues and substance abuse in order to help our clients and loved ones heal and have a chance to recover, however they define that for themselves.

SEXUALITY EDUCATION IN THE UNITED STATES

Sexuality encompasses the sexual knowledge, beliefs, feelings, attitudes, values, intentions, and behavior of individuals as well as sensuality, intimacy, sexual identity, and sexual health (Sexuality Information and Education Council of the United States, 1990). Too often, both the formal and the informal sexuality education that an individual receives in our society is inaccurate, fragmented, and diminished as well as biased and incomplete (Sears, 1992). There is no better example of the toll this negative sexuality education has taken than for people in treatment for substance abuse. In order for men and women to recover, they need to believe that something in their world makes sense and has real meaning. Incorporating learning in a way that makes sense to the learner can have positive results in real life. Relating subject matter to these clients' interests, needs, and experiences allows them to attach personal meaning to the learning. According to La Cursia, Beyer, and Ogletree (1994), "a sexuality education philosophy should reflect the 'real life' experiences and needs of students." In order to determine the specific sexuality needs of people in treatment, an exploration of how they perceive their sexuality is warranted.

Negative Views of Sex

It is the norm in U.S. culture to grow up with negative sexual scripts that purport a moderate sexual drive, monogamous (often married and heterosexual) relationships, limited sexual experience, and procreative sex (Levine & Troiden, 1988). In sex-negative societies, any kind of sexuality that occurs outside the norm is then seen as deviant or abnormal. Other cultures have more sex-positive stances, where what is seen in U.S. culture as deviant is normal and healthy for them. So what define sexual behaviors as deviant are *not* actually the behaviors themselves but rather *how the society one lives in perceives and judges these behaviors.*

Defining sexual behaviors as deviant may create cognitive dissonance (confusion) within individuals with regard to how they perceive their own sexual desire and behavior, which can lead one to believe that their sexuality is "out of control" or inherently bad (Stevenson, 1996).

Reinforcing a negative belief can be counterproductive to the recovery process if it results in shame-based thinking. The internalization of what is deemed healthy (through societal norms, religion, politics, and education) becomes the mechanism that causes the distress in individuals as they develop and attempt to form relationships based on limited options for perceived "normal" sexual functioning. This phenomenon, coupled with substance abuse, creates a pattern of self-destructive behavior (sexual and otherwise) that contributes to the downward spiral that addiction results in.

A HOLISTIC APPROACH TO SEXUAL HEALTH

Teaching about sexuality from a holistic approach, including areas that are not typically taught in health education classes, family, or religion, becomes important and necessary. Traditionally, what gets covered (if at all) in school relates primarily to the blue-light special. This is the area of sexual health and reproduction and covers topic areas of reproductive anatomy, disease prevention, health issues and concerns, birth control, and reproductive options (Kirby, 2000). It is the "nuts and bolts" of sexuality. Yet many programs are not allowed to cover many of the basics with the oppression that abstinence-only curricula bring. This leaves people without the accurate information and resources needed to make informed choices regarding their sexual health and sexuality. It is a barrier to developing healthy sexuality.

Areas of sexuality that are often not included in sexuality-related programming are those that include issues of sensuality, sexual identity, attitudes and feelings, and sexualization. These areas, for many, are the areas that cause them shame, confusion, trauma, low self-esteem, poor body image, eating disorders, self-hatred, homophobia, sexual dysfunction, poor communication skills, failed relationships, and more. It is these topics that are covered in more depth as we move around the circles of sexuality with regard to enhancing recovery from addiction.

What is sexual health? The World Health Organization (WHO, 1975) defines sexual health using the following framework:

Sexual health is an approach to sexuality founded in accurate knowledge, personal awareness and self-acceptance, such that one's behavior, values, and emotions are congruent and integrated within a person's wider personality structure and self-definition. Sexual health involves an ability to be intimate with a partner, to communicate explicitly about sexual needs and desires, to be sexually

functional (to have desire, become aroused, and obtain sexual fulfill-
ment), to act intentionally and responsibly, and to set appropriate
sexual boundaries. Sexual health has a communal aspect, reflecting
not only self-acceptance and respect, but also respect and appre-
ciation for individual differences and diversity, as well as a feeling
of belonging to and involvement in one's own sexual culture(s). Sexual health includes a sense of self-esteem, personal attractiveness,
and competence, as well as freedom from sexual dysfunction, sexually transmitted diseases, and sexual assault and coercion. Sexual
health affirms sexuality as a positive force, enhancing other dimensions of one's life. (Robinson, Bockting, Rosser, Miner, & Coleman,
2002, p. 45)

Each of the circles in Sexual Beingness has its own set of characteristics
based on gender, age, race, culture, experience, and so on. Based on these
topic areas within the circles, content is first explained in a general knowledge base, then in relation to substance abuse and recovery issues. Each
chapter examines each topic and includes methods of teaching about these
issues in the treatment realm. The scope of this book does not allow for in-
depth study of each issue, so resources to obtain more information are
included at the end of each chapter.

Terminology

Next, there is a considerable amount of terminology that may be unfa-
miliar or confusing. I try to address some of these terms in more detail
in the chapters that make most sense to define them in. The only circle
where "the facts" will not be covered in great detail in this book is the
blue-light special. Any undergraduate textbook on human sexuality covers this in explicit detail. Issues related to the blue-light special are discussed in relation to feelings and attitudes to sexually transmitted
infection/HIV risk behaviors and harm reduction as well as sexual functioning. These are also areas that can trigger relapse in people with
substance use issues.

SEXUAL SELF-ESTEEM

Sexual what? We have all heard about self-esteem—a person's self-
perceptions of him- or herself. Sexual self-esteem has to do with a
person's perceptions of how good he or she feels (or doesn't) about him-
or herself as a sexual being. This concept is relatively new in the research

realm, with some of the early studies being done in the late 1980s and early 1990s. As a graduate student, I became intrigued by the concept as it related to substance abusers. Did people with substance abuse and sexual problems have lower sexual self-esteem than people who had less abusive pasts? Could sexual self-esteem function as a measure of sexual health in recovery and the treatment process? Would increasing sexual self-esteem improve treatment outcomes? Much of my academic study and research thus far has centered on attempting to answer some of these questions, with some promising results.

The concept of sexual self-esteem is relatively recent and understudied. Gaynor and Underwood (1995) describe sexual self-esteem as "the tendency to value, versus devalue, one's own sexuality, thereby being able to approach rather than avoid sexual experiences both with self and others" (p. 334). These authors note that family background, peer group influence, and personal experience all contribute to acquiring positive or negative sexual self-esteem. Zeanah and Schwarz (1996) define sexual self-esteem as "one's affective reactions to one's sexual thoughts, feelings and behaviors" (p. 3). These researchers maintain that in order to effectively link self-perceptions with sexual behaviors, the affective realm of individual's cognitive appraisals (or thought processes) must be addressed in the sexual domain. Affective realms refer to the individual's feeling good or bad as a result of these cognitive appraisals. Positive reactions include feelings of pride, satisfaction, or security. Negative feelings might include disappointment, dissatisfaction, confusion, or a sense of vulnerability or insecurity.

SEXUAL SELF-ESTEEM IN RECOVERY

Sexual self-esteem appears to be a distinguishable aspect of sexuality and as a result may offer a promising focus for identifying possible links between sexuality and the recovery process for substance-abusing individuals. These links include relapse triggers, such as past sexual abuse or sexual assault, risky sexual behavior, sexual orientation, low body image, and sexual dysfunction, to name a few. If individuals have acquired negative sexual self-esteem, this may contribute to their substance abuse, addiction, and relapse if not addressed in treatment. Damaged sexual self-esteem can be viewed as a type of disability and has also been linked with sexual revictimization and child sexual abuse (Mayers, Heller, & Heller, 2003; Van Bruggen, Runtz, & Kadlec, 2006). Exploring the etiology of low sexual self-esteem in substance-abusing clients may provide new links for future treatment interventions.

I am currently developing a specialized sexual health psychoeducational curriculum for women in substance abuse treatment based on the results of several studies that have examined the sexuality links related to recovery, substance abuse, and sexual self-esteem. Although the current research has centered on the use of sexual self-esteem and women, there is certainly room for exploration of the concept with men as well. In 2007, I developed, tested, and validated a shortened version consisting of 27 items and have found similar results in my current research utilizing the shortened measure. The revised measure examines five separate domains of sexuality: sexual satisfaction, body image, sexual skill/efficacy, sexual regret/shame, and sexual control. Each of these domains measures areas that are included in the Sexual Beingness model, and all were found to be significantly correlated with substance use and sexuality connections in my research thus far.

Sexual Satisfaction

Sexual Satisfaction subscale items are consistent with self-perceptions of feeling satisfied with one's sex life. Scores on the scale range from 6 to 30, with low scores indicating personal dissatisfaction with one's relationship to one's personal sex life. Items directly reflect the concept of sexual satisfaction. Lawrance and Byers (1995) described sexual satisfaction as "an affective response arising from one's subjective evaluation of the positive and negative dimensions associated with one's sexual relationship" (p. 268). The measurement of this "affective response" is not necessarily a simple task. The use of a multi-item scale allows the researcher to consider various components or dimensions of a sexual relationship. This approach may provide a more accurate reflection of a person's overall satisfaction with his or her sexual relationship than would approaches that used only one or two items (Young, Luquis, Denny, & Young, 1998).

Body Image

The Body Image subscale items are directly correlated to an individual's perceptions of body image, how one feels about one's appearance, and personal desires to "look better." Scores on the scale range from 6 to 30, with low scores indicating dissatisfaction with one's views of one's body, looks, or weight. Body image has been researched with regard to sexual self-esteem, substance use, and disordered eating. Eating disorders are related to body image and are included in sexual health models (Advocates for Youth, 2011; Robinson et al., 2002). It has been well documented that women are objectified more than men: "Women's bodies are looked at, evaluated, and always potentially objectified" (Fredrickson & Roberts, 1997, p. 175). Correspondingly, men place greater emphasis on a potential mate's physical attractiveness than do women (Buss, 1994; Feingold, 1992). Self-consciousness over one's sexual attractiveness may be a mediating factor in relationships between women's body size, body image, and heterosexual experience. According to a study on sexual-esteem and body image among young college women, "it appears that sexual-esteem for a woman is at least partially based on a sense of confidence in her own physical attractiveness" (Weiderman & Hurst, 1998, p. 279). Qualitative studies suggest that body size and body image play important roles in the sexuality of women and that body size and body image may interact with certain characteristics of women's intimate relationship partners (Daniluk, 1993). Men are impacted by body image in similar ways, being expected to be tough and masculine, so having a muscular body is a myth that men fall prey to, both straight and gay. Steroid use and compulsive behavior to achieve an unrealistic physical image can negatively affect men. This will be explored in more depth in Chapter 7.

Sexual Skill/Efficacy

The Sexual Skill/Efficacy subscale items describe one's perceived sexual skill and ability to effectively please a sexual partner and one's self-efficacy in communicating in a sexual situation. Previous research with the original scale has consistently found that women with more sexual experience score higher on the original Skill/Experience subscale (Shapiro & Schwarz, 1997; Zeanah & Schwarz, 1996). The perceived ability to communicate around sexual issues is an important aspect of a healthy noncoercive relationship (Braun-Harvey, 2009). Including efficacy as part of the perceived skill base may help measure improvement in communication skill for women in relationships where her power has been diminished. Scores range from 5 to 25 on this scale, with low score representing a diminished perception of ability to effectively please a partner, ability to communicate sexual needs, and feel good at sex in a relationship.

Sexual Regret/Shame

Sexual Regret/Shame subscale items describe one's perceived sexual morality and guilt, specifically guilt and shame associated with sexual activities that are not congruent with one's self-defined morals and standards. Feeling guilt and shame about sexual activities has been linked in part to religious values and can cause a great deal of personal angst for women and men as they explore sexual behaviors that may go against their

BRIEF SEXUAL SELF-ESTEEM INVENTORY FOR WOMEN
Revised by
Raven James, PhD, and Lori Simons, PhD

Instructions—Please read carefully:

You are asked to rate your feelings about several aspects of sexuality. You are not asked to describe your actual experiences but to rate your reactions and feelings about your experiences, whatever they may be. In this questionnaire, "sex" and "sexual activity" refer to a variety of sexual behaviors, including hugging, kissing, caressing, and petting, as well as sexual intercourse. Current sexual activity is not necessary in order to answer the questions. There are no right or wrong answers; reactions to and feelings about sexuality are normally quite varied. What is important are your reactions to your own personal experiences, thoughts, and feelings.

Please answer each questions as honestly as possible. Using the rating scale at the top of each page, place the number which most closely matches the way you feel to the left of the question.

1	2	3	4	5	6
Strongly Disagree	Moderately Disagree	Mildly Disagree	Mildly Agree	Moderately Agree	Strongly Agree

____ 1.   I am happy about my sex life.

____ 2.   I like my body.

____ 3.   I worry that I won't be able to stop doing something I don't want to in a sexual situation.

____ 4.   I never feel bad about my sexual behaviors.

____ 5.   All in all, I feel satisfied with my sex life.

____ 6.   I feel disappointed with my sex life.

____ 7.   I am happy with the way I look.

____ 8.   I feel okay about telling my partner what I want in a sexual situation.

____ 9.   Some of the things I do in sexual situations are morally wrong.

____ 10.   I am where I want to be sexually, at this point in my life.

____ 11.   I feel that "sexual techniques" come easily to me.

____ 12.   I hate my body.

____ 13.   I am afraid of losing control sexually.

____ 14.   I never feel guilty about my sexual feelings.

____ 15.   I feel good about the place of sex in my life.

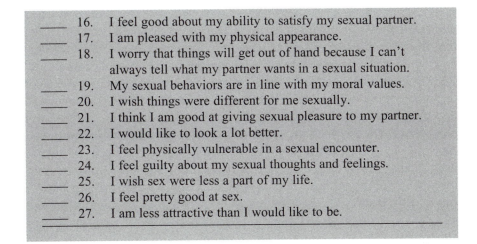

religious upbringing. Internalizing this shame can be problematic for a number of reasons, including damage resulting from self-blame over sexual abuse and nonconsensual sexual events as well as sexual revictimization (Braun-Harvey, 2009; James, 2011; Runtz, 2003; Shapiro & Schwarz, 1996). Scores range from 6 to 30 on this scale, with low scores representing a high level of sexual guilt and shame and high scores representing a perceived feeling of congruence with sexual behaviors and self-defined morals.

Sexual Control

Sexual Control subscale items describe one's perceived ability to feel in control of sexual situations with a partner. Sexual attachment models support a claim of fearful attachment and its subsequent results associated with worry over control in relationships and tendencies to be anxious, fearful, and unassertive when it comes to sexual relationships (Bartholomew & Horowitz, 1991; Feeney & Noller, 1996). This type of attachment in the revised sexual self-esteem scale explains the relationship of these factor items related to sexual control. Scores range from 4 to 20 on this scale, with low scores representing a high level of anxiety and fear over perceived control in sexual relationships and high scores representing one's ability to assert oneself in a sexual relationship with confidence.

CONSIDERING TREATMENT OUTCOMES

In terms of providing sexual health interventions for people in treatment (or any other intervention for that matter), being able to measure outcomes is important. If we can't measure it, we don't know if it works. When I worked in HIV/substance use, we measured and tracked everything we did, from the number of trainings we provided to the makeup of participants (gender and ethnicity) and behavior change as a result of participation in programs. In order to provide comprehensive services, we need to be able to say that we did what we said we would do. Agencies are accountable to their funders, and being able to provide effective services also means that agencies are more competitive for grants and continued funding. As sexual self-esteem continues to measure improved sexual health outcomes, it can be utilized as one method for measuring program outcomes. So, if one of our sexual health outcomes states that clients will improve their sexual self-esteem, we will be able to measure this through a pretest/posttest using the measure (prior to a sexual health group and after). In these economic times, positive outcome evaluation can be critical to the survival for some agencies. The construct of sexual self-esteem is discussed throughout the remaining chapters as it relates to measuring outcomes and its relevance to current findings connected to substance abuse. Of course, there are many other measurement tools available for specific topics, such as HIV risk, sexual risk-reduction, self-efficacy around sexual communication, and so in. More of these are introduced and defined in the chapters they most relate to.

SEXUALITY ATTITUDE REASSESSMENT TRAINING

For almost 40 years, SAR workshops have been offered to tens of thousands of participants around the United States in order to educate health professionals, medical students, clergy, doctors, and the general public about sexuality across the life span, sexual ethics and morals, sexual variations, sexuality and physical disabilities, sexual orientation, negative sexual experiences, and masturbation (Halstead & Halstead, 1983; Held, Cournoyer, Held, & Chilgren, 1974; Rosser et al., 1995; Stayton, 1998; Wollert, 1978). "Their dual purpose is to promote an increased understanding of participants' own sexuality and to help participants analyze their attitudes toward the sexuality of others. The main difference between SAR education and typical sexuality education courses is the use of sexually explicit media which are gradually introduced using systematic principles of desensitization" (Robinson et al., 2002, p. 45). These materials help participants in clarifying their responses to sex and sexuality, alleviating shame and enhancing comfort. Of course, facilitator experience in managing group affect is critical in this type of training. I highly recommend a SAR to any professional who will be working with sexuality issues in order for them to become immersed in experiential learning. Having the SAR experience enables professionals to understand the sensitive nature of teaching about sexuality in a group setting and provides a solid base from which to work.

NEXT STEPS

Now that we having a working model for sexuality-related issues and a framework in which to conceptualize them, we will want to consider how we will go about discussing sexual matters in our respective programs or practices. Having all the knowledge in the world won't do us much good unless we have established a sense of personal comfort and can communicate with clients. So, now let's talk about sex!

RESOURCES

Books

Braun-Harvey, D. (2011). *Sexual health in recovery: A professional counselor's manual.* New York: Springer.

Weiss, K. E. (2010). *SAR Sexual Attitude Reassessment seminars: A retrospective of SAR early years in Minnesota.* Minneapolis: Itasca Books.

Online Resource

Advocates for Youth. http://www.advocatesforyouth.org

TWO

Sex Talk

My mother used to say, "If you don't have anything nice to say, then don't say anything at all."

—Anonymous

I used to joke that I was a sex worker—I talked about sex and got paid for it. But talking about sex is no joking matter. That's about as safe as we can get with regard to sexual risk: talk about it. Sexual communication is one of the biggest factors in negotiating relationships, intimacy, safer sex, values, behaviors, and sexual desires. If we aren't able to say the words, name the behaviors, or correctly identify what we are trying to convey to a partner, we are at risk for potentially negative consequences. In U.S. culture, it seems the norm to talk about sex through the use of humor, and often the humor that accompanies the conversation has the brunt of some group as the punch line. I cannot even count the times I have heard people make fun of those whose sexual orientation and behaviors are different from their own, and this does not exclude health care providers or counselors.

IMPORTANCE OF LANGUAGE

Imagine a client in treatment who is lesbian, gay, bisexual, or transgender (LGBT) and in a therapy group. The group topic is about HIV prevention, a typical topic to be discussed in the course of treatment. The presenter is discussing sexual transmission, and one of the group members makes a disparaging comment about how HIV is about gay sex and they are not gay, so this has nothing to do with them. How the counselor responds or doesn't to the comment will have a lasting impact on everyone in that group, not just the LGBT client, who may or may not be "out" to the rest of the group members. The presenter has a few options: (1) he or she can ignore the comment (which tells the client and the rest of the group members that it is okay to bash LGBT people and that being LGBT will put them at risk for future shame and ridicule), (2) he or she can mistakenly collude with the group member and foster a negative and unsafe group experience, or (3) he or she can address the member's comments as inappropriate, provide rationale with correct information, and set boundaries around gay bashing in group, thus providing safety for LGBT clients and addressing inappropriate behavior through the use of language.

Talking about sex also involves utilizing appropriate language: language that promotes equality and safety. We may not want to think that a counselor would behave inappropriately with regard to sexual matters, but it happens more frequently than we would imagine. As a colleague, we would be a sexual health advocate to address sexist and heterosexist comments just as we would in terms of racism and other forms of oppression and discrimination. Learning how to advocate, what to say, how to say it, and how to follow through with consistency are skills that can be developed over time with practice.

Language can make us or break us when working with client groups. If we use terminology that is too technical or difficult to grasp, we may alienate or confuse clients. One philosophy involves the use of what I call "meeting clients where they are at." This is inclusive of culturally appropriate language. Being cognizant of clients' sexual language can help us achieve this goal. The use of mutual terminology can assist us in developing relationships that are based on equality and trust rather than an "us/them" mentality. If we do not understand the vernacular that clients are using to describe sexual acts, we need to ask. Sure, we are supposed to mentor, coach, and counsel, but if we are willing to listen and learn from the people we work with, our relationships will take on a whole new dimension of authenticity.

CLIENT RELUCTANCE

Take another scenario. This one involves a client who has had a risky sexual encounter and is embarrassed and fearful about what the consequences might be. This client desperately wishes to discuss the matter with their counselor and get advice on what to do in terms of testing for

sexually transmitted infections (STIs) and HIV and how to better negotiate condom use with future partners.

What might prevent this client from speaking to their counselor?
Possible reasons could include personal embarrassment, fear of being
judged, fear of violating one of the myths of early recovery, having a sexual relationship early on, not knowing how to bring it up, not wanting to
bring it up in a group setting, lacking knowledge of how to communicate,
and prior signals from the agency or counselor that sex is a "taboo" subject and is best avoided in terms of the client/counselor relationship.
Perhaps the client had tried to bring the subject up before (possibly in
another facility) and was "shut down" in terms of openly discussing sexual issues. Past negative experiences can inhibit clients from talking about
sexual matters in group or with their counselors.

Given this scenario, what might help a client feel able and willing to
discuss sexual matters? Possible solutions include an open, welcoming
environment within the agency setting. Do staff members routinely talk
about sex matter-of-factly in everyday conversations? Was a sexual history part of the client intake? Is there a sexual health group available at
the treatment center? What types of literature are made available (posters,
pamphlets, and so on)? Is STI/HIV test counseling routinely offered, and
are these services emphasized as part of the treatment process? Making
sexual health issues a part of treatment rather than apart from treatment
can create an environment that is conducive to positive sexual health in
treatment.

RELATIONSHIP CONSIDERATIONS

Commonly, situations arise with regard to sexual matters with health
care providers or friends, at meetings, or with family members. Personal
comfort is vital for discussion of sexual matters in relationships. The idea
of practice as progress can assist people in developing communication
comfort and skill. If you have never discussed sexual matters, you can
start at home with yourself. It may sound contrived, but like practicing a
speech in front of a mirror, talking about sex out loud to your mirror
may be the first step to developing comfort. For someone who has never
spoken the words "condom," "penis," "masturbation," or "vagina," utter-
ing the words aloud is the first step of the process.

Role playing or practicing "what-if" scenarios with a friend is another
method for developing comfort. I had a client once who was debating
whether to leave a relationship. She kept running reasons through her
mind about why she should stay versus why she should leave. I asked

her to write a list of reasons and to include the benefits of staying as well as the benefits of leaving, and then we talked about it next time she came in. Once she had written it down and then talked about the situation, her answers became clearer. Sometimes, the process of writing it down and then talking about it moves a person from the cognitive to the behavioral realm, and the issue loses its power. Clarity and critical thinking skills develop when we verbalize and reason with another person. To think that we are prepared for a relational encounter without having prepared is like showing up to give that speech without ever having rehearsed. Practice doesn't make us perfect, but it does make us better. We can prepare a scenario we are struggling with and role-play it, allowing us to devise potential responses for the encounter. Over time, we will develop a rationale and resolve to be prepared for numerous situations that we may have not considered on our own.

CREATING A POSITIVE, SAFE ENVIRONMENT

Clients come to counselors seeking support, knowledge, and care. Sexuality-related concerns often come up in treatment. When providing support to individuals around sexuality issues, care must be taken in order to be sensitive. Clients might be unable to talk about sexuality issues for fear of rejection, lack of safety, and embarrassment. Counselors can build positive relationships with clients by being open and nonjudgmental, allowing them to overcome their concerns of discussing sexuality. Clients may have concerns about issues such as unintended pregnancy, STIs, intimacy, abuse, or relationships. They may lack sexuality information, life skills, and knowledge of sexual health resources, and it is up to providers to be knowledgeable in sexual health matters. If providers are not able to discuss sexual matters, they should consider attending trainings to increase comfort around sexual issues.

The following guidelines are intended to develop a safe environment for sexual health conversations (this list is not exhaustive, but it does provide a starting place for conversation):

- Have sexual health material in waiting rooms, offices, and so on
- Have welcoming, diverse individuals on staff
- Do not make assumptions about client behaviors, sexual orientation, sexual identity, relationship status, or health status
- Do not assume that there is only one issue or that the presenting issue is necessarily what the client really wished to discuss

- Use nonjudgmental language and monitor nonverbal responses
- Do not judge clients for engaging in behavior that is not in line with your moral values or beliefs
- Use open-ended questions; let the client take the lead and encourage further exploration of issues
- Meet the client where they are at; do not force them to a solution that they do not want or agree on
- Explore the pros and cons of situations; let the client experience or struggle with their ambivalence over decisions (this can aid them in moving toward change)
- Ask about their expectations of the session and what they hope to achieve
- Be understanding and supportive
- Use language that the client understands
- If you do not understand terminology your client is using, ask him or her to explain it to you
- Be confident
- Respect clients' nondisclosure and privacy
- Be youth and "queer" positive: respect who the client is as an individual
- Use inclusive language (be familiar with terms of sexual diversity)
- Do not push your views on clients (i.e., abortion, abstinence, or religion)
- Make sure that the client knows that the support being provided is part of a collaborative process but that the final decision belongs to them
- Assist clients in developing plans for risk reduction and so on
- Provide relevant services, including referrals (adapted from Canadian Federation for Sexual Health, 2011)

Providing a safe environment for sexual health communication is only one piece of the larger picture. Other communication considerations include taking a sexual history as part of the intake and assessment process, having knowledgeable counselors on staff, providing sexuality groups for clients, knowledge of community resources for referral, and adequate training practices for new staff. A related issue is the inclusion of agency policies that reflect positive sexual health practices and that promote an environment that eliminates stigma and discrimination. Training new staff on inclusive policies is integral to fostering a positive and empowering climate.

TAKING A SEXUAL HISTORY

Conducting initial interviews with clients in treatment involves the use of an assessment tool called a biopsychosocial history. This tool is used in social work, counseling, mental health settings, and so on in order to get a holistic picture of a variety of components, past and present, that constitute an individual's life. Assessment includes medical history, family history, any psychiatric history, and demographic information. Some versions of assessment are more comprehensive than others; many do not routinely probe sexuality-related issues. Doctors and health providers do not always conduct in-depth sexual histories.

Reasons for not taking a sexual history include provider discomfort or embarrassment, lack of time, lack of knowledge, not feeling that it is important, and perceiving the client as not having the resources to pursue follow-up therapy. Sexual health is integral to overall health and well-being, so performing comprehensive sexual histories and assessing sexual health and functioning can enable providers to obtain pertinent information for prevention/intervention. Sexual health is a quality-of-life issue, and certain medications, illness, surgery, or other conditions can impact sexual functioning. Assessing these areas, in conjunction with proper training, enables providers to determine the impact of environment on sexual health issues. In addition, a sexual history provides information on sexual abuse, molestation, incest, rape, or other negative sexual experiences that may have impacted their substance use. We send strong messages to clients about how we value sexual health when we take the time to conduct comprehensive sexual histories. We also let clients know that we are willing to hear what they have to say and open the door for future conversations about sexuality, sexuality education, validating feelings, and directed client-centered sexuality counseling.

An important piece of conducting a sexual history centers on how we ask questions and what types of questions to ask. First, we should acknowledge the personal nature of the history. Most clients are accustomed to being asked about personal history but not necessarily specific sexual behaviors and practices. Normalizing the process is important, and using a blanket statement that assures them that you routinely assess these areas because they can impact sexual functioning and recovery efforts is one way to begin to normalize the assessment. Emphasizing confidentiality also helps establish client comfort. Always relate the questions to health and recovery to remind clients that you have their best interest in mind.

Next, issues to include on the sexual history can include the following:

- General health history
- Allergies (some people have latex allergies and cannot use latex condoms)
- Recent medication(s)
- Recent illness or surgeries
- Past STIs
- Women: brief gynecological history
- HIV risk factors (injection drug use and partner's status)
- HIV testing history
- Past and current sexual practices
- Gender of partners
- Number of partners
- Most recent sexual exposure
- New sex partners
- Patterns of condom use
- Partner's condition
- Substance abuse associated with sexual behavior
- Domestic violence issues (see Appendix A for sample sexual questionnaire)

TALKING ABOUT SEX

How to Ask

When I worked for the AIDS organization, we conducted comprehensive sexual histories with all our new clients. We utilized an interactive approach through the use of both open-ended and closed-ended questions and active listening to ensure that the session was responsive to an individual client's needs. Staff's best work came from maintaining a neutral approach and a nonjudgmental attitude. Counselors and therapists are typically trained to steer clear from using closed-ended questions, but they serve a purpose in taking a sexual history. In the event a client may be uncomfortable about sharing certain information, being flexible and using closed-ended questions can enable providers to elicit the information they need while respecting the client's privacy.

Avoid Assumptions

A provider's personal values and biases must not be allowed to interfere with the relationship with the client. Providers should never make assumptions about clients' sexual orientation, sexual practices, relationships, or substance use based on appearance, ethnicity, age, or other factors. Taking personal stock of our comfort zone with sexuality issues can assist us in identifying any biases we may have. I have yet to meet someone who is perfectly comfortable with every sexual subject under the sun. One way to begin this personal reflection is to take the Sexuality Comfort Self-Assessment (Appendix B).

The Sexuality Comfort Self-Assessment is designed to assist providers in examining their personal comfort with discussing specific sexuality topics and behaviors. Although there may be a number of areas you may not feel equipped to discuss, taking the personal assessment will help you identify areas that you can develop more knowledge about and comfort in. It is preferable to know this information prior to conducting sexuality programming in order to better serve your clients. If a topic comes up that you are visibly uncomfortable with, you may lose credibility and rapport with your group.

It is important to begin your conversation using gender-neutral language that does not imply an assumption of heterosexuality. As part of the sexual history, specifically ask every client about the gender of their sex partner. Most patients do not object to answering questions about whether they have male or female partners or both, although they may not volunteer this information without being asked. If we ask about partner gender, we also open the door to a welcoming, safe environment. Some clients will play the "pronoun game," avoiding naming the sex of their partner but alluding to it through gender-neutral language.

Some clients understand anatomical and medical language, such as "vaginal sex," "anal sex," and "oral sex," but others do not, so be prepared to explain any terminology the client does not understand. The way in which we speak to clients should be tailored to the client's age, culture, and educational level, so it is imperative that staff receive some form of sexuality training, attend a Sexuality Attitude Reassessment, or become familiar with terminology through reading. As was mentioned earlier, if a client uses terminology we are not familiar with, we need to ask for clarification. If we are uncertain that language is culturally appropriate, check with the client to see if the language is acceptable. Asking permission and showing sensitivity to clients will help build trust and rapport.

Ask every client about current and past substance abuse; injection drug use in particular is a high risk factor for HIV infection. Substance abuse can put clients at risk for HIV infection in several other ways as well, including a compromised immune system (creates a more vulnerable host), exposure to or infection with other STIs, decreasing inhibitions, and blacking out (drinking to the point where there is no memory of behavior but a person can still function physically), or passing out (potential risk for sexual assault, common at large parties).

COMMUNICATION SKILLS

Nonverbal communication helps develop rapport and communicate genuine interest. Maintaining eye contact, nodding, and using silence when culturally appropriate can be important ways to communicate without talking.

Questioning can use a combination of open-ended and closed-ended questions to gather the information of a sexual history.

Open-ended questions are an important tool for effective sexual history taking. Open-ended questions are ones that cannot be answered with a yes-or-no answer. These questions usually start with "who," "what," "when," "where," or "how." Open-ended questions help people to open up, encourage more conversation, and give the client some degree of control over what he or she wants to share.

Closed-ended questions are effective when all that is needed is a yes-or-no answer or a specific piece of information, such as a date. These types of questions are also useful with a client who is particularly uncomfortable discussing these issues.

Acknowledge feelings to show an understanding of how the client feels. Ask questions that help the client explore his or her feelings in more detail. Many people need to have their feelings acknowledged and discussed before they are able to really *hear* information. Ignoring someone's feelings can damage or disrupt a sexual history-taking session.

Summarize what the client says to clarify information and to allow the client to judge whether you understood them correctly and then at the end of a session to review the client's plan of action (Center for Health Training, 2011).

Gaining Confidence

While the remaining chapters in this book address specific topics of sexuality, being able to gain confidence in communication and developing rapport with clients is critical, so in addition to incorporating sexuality issues through intake procedures, we also want to be able to facilitate sexuality groups. All people are sexual beings, and our substance-using clients are very likely to have experienced some component of Sexual Beingness that was connected to their use. By conducting sexual health histories, we gain opportunities to identify areas of sexual health that should be addressed in treatment. Whether we are considering developing or teaching a sexuality group in treatment, having some communication skills for group work is essential.

EXISTING CURRICULA

In addition to the lessons and ideas provided in this text, there are a number of sexuality-related programs for use in addiction treatment (or ones that include sexuality issues) that already exist (e.g., Braun-Harvey, 2009; Institute of Behavioral Research, 2011; Najavits, 2002). I encourage providers to explore already existing materials, assess client need, and use your judgment to decide which particular topics your clients may benefit from and when.

Although the need for sexual health–related programming in the treatment domain is not new, it has not yet been nationally recognized as a standard of treatment. Many agencies and counselors have been addressing sexuality in treatment for years. Recent developments in treating sexual health issues in addiction have continued to move the issue to the forefront of the field (Braun-Harvey, 2009, 2011; James, 2011). Constructing effective programs can involve years of planning, piloting, testing, evaluating, and refining. As such, this area is in its relative infancy in terms of rigorous scientific research trials.

ADDRESSING RESISTANCE AND PERSONAL BIAS

Barriers to communicating about sex with clients, as well as approaches and communication skills, are similar to those described for taking a sexual history. Evaluating personal comfort, values clarification, and identifying provider bias are essential. The following information and activities will expose you to several methods of exploring sexual communication with clients. One important thing to keep in mind when facilitating sexuality groups is that we, as facilitators, will continue to be challenged by client reactions and clashes with our own personal bias and values.

An example of this was when I was learning how to facilitate HIV overviews to client groups in drug and alcohol treatment centers in upstate

New York. I had conducted many programs on my own, but on this particular occasion my supervisor was tagging along to evaluate my progress. It was an outpatient program, and I had a group of about 25 clients, most of whom were men. I had 60 minutes with this group, which was shorter than a typical 90-minute session. While discussing transmission, one of the men raised his hand and asked, "Where did HIV come from?" He was an African American man, and I launched into an explanation of some of the HIV origin theories, which included examples of mutation from chimpanzees in Africa as well as government conspiracy theory and racial genocide. After about five minutes, more people chimed in. The group successfully derailed me from finishing on time, and when time was up, people started to get up and leave while I was still trying to get through the material.

Needless to say, I was extremely frustrated and embarrassed as well as anxious and stressed about the fact I was being evaluated on such a poor performance (in my eyes). On the ride home, she matter-of-factly pointed out some observations of how the group wrested control from me and provided some suggestions on how to effectively get them back on track in those situations. One of the suggestions she gave me that I still use today is to provide information, validate what the participant has said, move the group on by stating that there is more information to cover, and let them know that if they want to discuss the topic in more depth after the program, I will be available to do so. Often participants challenge material not necessarily because they want to learn more but for other reasons, such as personal discomfort. If a situation such as this arises, make sure that you attend to the person(s) in question following the session to check in and maintain rapport. If you say you will be available after and then you disappear, you lose credibility with the group.

Learning how to manage emotional reactions, challenging behaviors, and heated discussions is a skill that we develop over time with practice. It is simpler to manage one person's reactions (with taking sexual histories) than to manage a whole group of people. Do not be discouraged if you have occasional setbacks; this is normal. With proper supervision and continual self-reevaluation, you will improve and become more comfortable with resistance and handling sensitive issues. I have never had this situation repeat itself (not being able to keep the group on task), but one of the lessons I learned was that, as a facilitator, I needed to develop what I call "crowd-control" techniques in order to manage unrest. The other lesson involved how important supervision and evaluation were in allowing me as a facilitator to be effective, improve my techniques, and learn new skills. Teaching about sexuality is hard work. It is also integral to the recovery process, rewarding, and worth every minute we invest into the process.

SEXUAL COMMUNICATION TIP

When teaching sexuality groups, the first critical component to address is group guidelines. In the thousands of client groups I have facilitated over the years, I discovered that setting guidelines from the outset can help prevent many problems later on, whether you meet once or over several months. Community health educators and group facilitators need to have a number of materials at their disposal. The most important ones are fresh markers (permanent and dry erase), butcher block paper or newsprint, and masking tape. Some group rooms are equipped with dry erase whiteboards or easels. Prepare newsprint ahead (or write on the whiteboard) and label your page "group guidelines." After providing an introduction to your topic (HIV overview, relationships, intimacy, and so on), stress to the group the need for respect and appropriate behavior and create this climate through the use of setting guidelines they wish to include. Eliciting responses from group members, write their responses on the paper, making sure to discuss the relevance as the ideas are brainstormed. If this is an open-ended group where clients enter and leave at differing points in time, you can create your own guidelines ahead of time, making sure that each client receives a copy prior to joining the group and that each agrees to abide by the guidelines while a member of the group.

Having guidelines allows that group leader to address any violations, if they occur, within the group setting. Having group guidelines mean that the facilitator has the responsibility to keep the group on task. If guidelines are violated, the manner in which the leader addresses them is important. Gentle reminders of mutual respect are the most appropriate method. We want to make sure we do not treat clients punitively for making mistakes, as the nature of being human is to err. For example, a client consistently interrupts other clients or makes inappropriate comments about a group of people. The facilitator's response might resemble the following: "Remember when we agreed that only one person would share at a time?" Physically posting guidelines in the group room and pointing to the item in question, respect, and repeating it is another tactic. Gentle yet assertive approaches to guideline violations also establish our credibility as a leader who is respectful and trustworthy.

SAMPLE SEXUALITY LESSON FOR AN INTRODUCTORY SESSION

Goal: Participants will be introduced to the curriculum and begin to develop comfort in communicating about sexuality issues.
Rationale: Sexuality is often perceived by learners as embarrassing, private, and potentially traumatizing. Setting up the introduction to the

curriculum and brainstorming ground rules provides reassurance for many learners (Bruess & Greenberg, 2004). Ground rules also provide for boundaries, which in turn facilitate a sense of safety within a group. By using learning activities that have low risk-taking levels, participants are gently guided into thinking and talking about sexuality issues. Similar to the foundation of a house, it must be solid enough to support the rest of the structure.

Time: 90 minutes
Objectives: Participants will do the following:

- Develop group guidelines
- Identify two sources of why discussing sexuality is difficult or uncomfortable
- Determine which sexuality issues are connected to their substance use

Materials:

- Blank newsprint paper for brainstorming group guidelines
- Blank index cards
- Container for collecting index cards
- Two prepared newsprint sheets, one labeled "fear/anxiety" and one labeled "something I want to learn." These sheets should be hanging on the wall before participants enter the room, folded up halfway so the headings cannot be seen.
- A list of sentence completions for journal ideas
- Sexual Beingness sheets (Figure 1.1 in Chapter 1)
- Markers and pens
- Journals

Introduction (25 minutes):
Facilitator self-introduces and then discusses purpose of the program, relating content to the recovery process and relapse prevention. Ask participants to self-introduce and say why they are in class (attendance may or may not be voluntary). Give an overview so that they know what to expect. Thank them for attending.

Hand out one index card to each participant. Ask them to write something they would like to learn from this program on one side of the card and a fear or anxiety they have about participating on the other side.

Instruct them to *not* write their names on the cards. Unveil the prepared, prelabeled sheets so they have the added visual of instructions and allow a few minutes to write down responses. When they are finished, collect the cards and place them in the container. Pass the container around the group and instruct them to take one card out of the container. Tell them they should not have their own card but, if they do, that no one in the group will know. One by one, go around the room and ask them to read off responses from the card they have. The facilitator should write those responses down on the appropriate newsprint.

The facilitator should now process the responses on the "fear/anxiety" sheet. Tell them that these fears and anxieties are normal and that we will address some of them by developing our guidelines. Also inform them that part of the reason for doing this exercise is so that they can see what fears other participants may have, that some of the fears are similar, and that by seeing them, we can, as a group, respect anxieties someone may have about participating. By normalizing fears, we reduce anxiety in the group. Tell them to consider this when they experience strong emotion to an issue that may come up for them. The facilitator should read off what is on the "what I want to learn" sheet and let the participants know which of their responses will be addressed (or not) in this curriculum.

Briefly discuss the importance of guidelines (see communication tip) and facilitate a brainstorm, eliciting responses from the group. The facilitator should record participant responses on the newsprint and make sure the following are listed:

- Encourage participants to express themselves honestly
- Ask that confidentiality be respected
- Urge risk taking
- Expect participation from everyone
- Punctuality (Silberman, 2006)

Once guidelines are complete, the facilitator should process each one to make sure the group understands why they are there and agree to have them there. Guidelines should be posted on the wall during each group. The facilitator must remind members to adhere to guidelines if any violations occur throughout the program.

Parallel Lines Activity (20 minutes)
Have the group count off by twos. If there are an odd number of participants, the facilitator can be part of a group (or have the odd person observe).

Instruct each group to line up in front of each other so they are parallel to each other. Tell them they are line A and line B. Instruct them that you will read off each question and that line A will answer to line B. Line B is to listen but not respond verbally. Time them for approximately 90 seconds to two minutes for each response. Once line A has spoken, reread the question but instruct line B to talk to line A, with line A to listen.

Once each pair has answered the question, ask the person at the end of line A to rotate to the front of the line so that, for each new question, there are new participants speaking to each other. Keep your eye on time while they are speaking, and about 10 seconds before time is up, state loudly, "Take about 10 seconds and finish up!" At the 90-second mark, use verbal cues to bring the group's attention to you and then ask the person at the end of line A to rotate. Process the rest of the questions using this procedure. The facilitator should also be observing the reactions of participants as they answer the questions. Do they get quiet? Do they seem animated? Are they embarrassed? Can they speak for the whole 90 seconds? Use this observation to process the discussion afterward.

Sample Questions:

1. What did you have for dinner last night?
2. Describe the street you grew up on.
3. What did you learn about sexuality from your parents?
4. What did you learn about sexuality growing up from your peers?
5. What did you learn about sexuality growing up from your church or spirituality?
6. What does the term "healthy sexuality" mean to you?

After completing the activity, ask the group members to return to their seats.

Follow-Up/Discussion (15 minutes):
Ask participants the following questions, interjecting your observations of how they reacted to certain questions during processing:

- What did it feel like to do this activity?
- Were any of the questions difficult to talk about? If so, which ones and why?
- Why do you think it is important to have this discussion?
- Do you think any of the topics relate to your addiction? How and why?

Sexual Beingness—An Overview (15 minutes):
Distribute the Sexual Beingness sheet. Provide information on the sexuality model and explain each circle and its relation to addiction/recovery. Ask for volunteers (in case someone has trouble reading and wishes not to be identified) to read off the topic of a circle and the descriptors underneath it. Begin with the "getting to know you" circle, and after someone reads it, spend a few minutes describing what the circle means in terms of application to relationships. Go clockwise around the sheet, using the same method to briefly cover each area.

Once the circles are introduced, inform the group that we will cover some of the areas in the circles throughout the program, and each session will examine different aspects of Sexual Beingness. Each subsequent session will cover areas under the topics in more depth as we move clockwise around the circles, looking at each aspect of the model until all areas have been explored. Ask for questions or comments before moving on to the next exercise.

Wrap-Up and Evaluation (10 minutes):
Hand out an extra copy of Sexual Beingness and ask them to circle areas within the circles that they feel are related to their own substance use. On the back of the sheets, ask them to write down two reasons they think talking about sexuality is difficult. Collect the sheets afterward.

Distribute journals to each group member. Inform them that each week, short homework assignments will be given and that they should use their journals as a place to record their reflections on the material presented in group. Ask participants to use the sentence completions as a jump-start for journaling. Ask them to write a few paragraphs on thoughts or feelings they had concerning the learning and/or sentence completions. Each subsequent lesson begins by voluntary sharing of journal entries to follow up from the previous week and/or to address any concerns. Ask if they have any questions about the program and clarify any confusion before concluding.

SENTENCE COMPLETIONS FOR JOURNALING IDEAS, WEEK 1

Sexuality to me is . . .
Sexual Beingness means . . .
Sexuality and addiction are . . .
The aspect of sexuality I feel is most connected to my substance use is . . .

NEXT STEPS

Talking about sex can create anxiety in our clients as well as providers. The importance of understanding our feelings and attitudes toward behaviors and sexual terminology can help us learn how to approach clients with increased levels of sensitivity. Speaking of terminology, probably the most confusing definitions for folks, given the heterosexist society we live in, have to do with gender identity and sexual orientation, so we will continue our journey around the circles and make the next stop at sexual identity. See you there!

COMMUNICATION RESOURCES

Books

Bennett, L., & Holczer, G. (2010). *Finding and revealing your sexual self: A guide to communicating about sex.* New York: Rowman & Littlefield.

Guerrero, L. K., Anderson, P. A., & Walid, A. A. (2010). *Close encounters: Communication in relationships.* Thousand Oaks, CA: Sage.

Online Resources

Center for Growth, Inc. http://www.sextherapyinphiladelphia.com/index.htm

National Center for Biotechnology Information. (2009). *Sexual communication, sexual goals, and students' transition to college: Implications for sexual assault, decision-making, and risky behaviors.* http://www.ncbi.nlm.nih.gov/pmc/articles/PMC2874912.

THREE

Sexual Identity for Geeks

Be who you are and say what you feel, because those who mind don't matter and those who matter don't mind.

—Dr. Seuss

When we begin to conceptualize identity in general, many issues come into play, including race, culture, family of origin, religion, sexual orientation, and age, to name a few. The beauty of identity is that there are endless facets of being that make up our individual personalities—some negative, some positive—but all take on unique meaning for us as we develop and progress on our journey through life. Within those aspects of identity are subcultures that further define those aspects with more clarity. The dark side of identity *is what society has constructed* in terms of what is and is not valued culturally. This side of identity is what can lead to substance misuse when specific social and environmental factors interact to create vulnerability and risk.

For example, as an African American substance-using lesbian, there are many aspects of her unique being that are defined by the subcultures attached to them. Being African American incorporates a culture of pride, oppression, religious affiliation, political views, and much more. Just her race and gender speak worlds about who she is. Being female in U.S. society brings to mind certain images and stereotypes, and being an African American woman adds new images and stereotypes. Add a substance use problem, which has its own unique subculture, depending on her drug of choice, using history, method of use, and socioeconomic background.

If she grew up in poverty, she may have started using because of environmental risk factors. Opiate and heroin use bring with it specific methods of using; does she snort or shoot up, and what does she do to support her habit? Having a lesbian orientation adds yet another layer of complexities, including engagement in the bar scene and/or gender role variations that accompany her lifestyle (drag king, femme/butch, and so on). Along with her sexual orientation will be a unique set of circumstances based on family of origin, religion, and culture that shape how she feels about herself as a lesbian. She may be closeted to others, depending on the level of safety or support around her stage of sexual identity development. This is not an exhaustive description of the interplay between multiple identities by any means, nor does it include myriad other aspects of her identity. Human beings are complex and more so in terms of sexual identity and its impact on development.

DEFINING SEXUAL IDENTITY TERMINOLOGY

Before we venture any further, let's begin to define some terminology related to sexual identity. I say *begin* to define because defining terminology can (1) be personal, (2) change over time, (3) be defined differently by different groups of individuals, and (4) incorporate discussion and processing of this information. That being said, sexual identity is the sense of who a person is with regard to their birth sex and gender. One of my favorite handouts is titled "The Gender Umbrella." This handout is a neat conceptualization of what gender, gender role, and gender identity entail (see Figure 3.1).

A person who is intersex (formerly referred to as a hermaphrodite) is born with variable genitalia that may have both "male" and "female" components. Certain characteristics can be linked to the variety of chromosomal combinations other than the XX female and XY male combinations. These chromosomal and biological variations can create a variety of genital, hormonal, and developmental characteristics that defy traditional definitions of sex and gender. Intersexuals have bodies that transgress our culture's expectations of sex. These individuals may or may not transgress the gender role that they are assigned at birth. Some intersexual children are assigned a sex by the family medical doctor and are forced to undergo hormonal and/or surgical procedures in order to help create congruency with the assigned sex to theoretically help the child "fit in" to societal norms of gender and gender role. There are many problems associated with forcing gender assignment too early in life, and a great number of intersexual people have difficulties adjusting or feeling comfortable in

Figure 3.1   Adapted from the Center for Crime Victims and Sexual Assault.

Everyone Fits Under

The Gender Umbrella

Transgender refers to anyone who transgresses the gender role assigned to a member of his or her birth sex. A gender role consists of the attitudes, behaviors, appearances, and other characteristics culturally associated with one birth sex or another.

Man/Woman

- A person whose gender identity and expression are congruent with his or her birth sex, as defined by culture and society

"Drag"   Cross-dresser

- A man or women who, on occasion, dresses as a member of a different sex for the purpose of political/social activism, humor or entertainment

Transvestite

- A person who dresses in clothing generally regarded as appropriate for another gender, in well-defined and restricted circumstances. Most often, transvestites are heterosexual men who are married with children

Adrogyne

- An individual who may be comfortable in either male or female gender roles, and who is not committed to one or the other. Is often displayed through "gender expression".

Transgenderist Transgender Person

- One who's self-perception incorporates a range of human characteristics (including those labeled as both masculine and feminine) to achieve a "wholness" that cannot be attained within the confines of one gender

Non-Operative Transsexual or Gender Queer

- A person who lives fully as a member of a sex that is presumed to be incongruent with his or her birth genitalia, who does not opt to take hormones and/or undergo surgery

Pre/Post Operative Transsexual

- A person who lives fully as a member of a sex that is presumed to be incongruent with his or her birth genitalia, who opts to take hormones and/or undergo surgery as part of the transistion, or a combination of hormones/surgery the gender they were assigned. As a society, we often have trouble with ambiguity, so if people cannot categorize or label each other, those people who do not fit in the "accepted" identity box are often misunderstood and subsequently stigmatized. This fear of groups of people who do not fit culturally accepted "norms" has resulted in a historical climate of intolerance, prejudice, and persecution. More about this later.

Alphabet Soup

Alphabet soup is next: LGBTQQIA and so on. Why all the letters? Face it, we love our acronyms. Lesbian, gay, bisexual, transgender, queer, questioning, intersexual, ally—when we start to discuss terms related to sexual identity, life can get downright confusing. On the other hand, when we are able to learn about the "what" and the "why," life begins to make more sense on its own terms. When I conduct trainings with drug and alcohol counselors on sexual identity, I often hear lamenting about the changing order of the letters. "I thought it was GLBT" or "Why do you put the L first?" are typical responses. The need for sensitivity and respect when dealing with others as well as the fact that this is not the only area in which information changes in terms of political correctness are part of my response. I personally put the "L" first rather than the "G" to advocate for lesbian invisibility. In the gay community, gay typically refers to men, where lesbians are gay women. When HIV entered the scene in the 1980s, the focus was more on gay men's behaviors than lesbians and heterosexuals. Lesbians were rendered invisible, and still today the Centers for Disease Control and Prevention recognizes HIV risk according to group, not specific sexual behavior. In order to bring visibility to more marginalized groups, I feel it is important to place them at the head of the acronym. The following descriptions provide more detailed definitions related to sex, gender, identity, and sexual orientation:

Sex, in this context, describes anatomy and, for our purposes specifically, genital and reproductive anatomy. If you have a penis, a scrotum, testicles, and a prostate and XY chromosomes, your sex is generally referred to as male. If you have a vagina, a labia, a clitoris, a uterus, and ovaries and XX chromosomes, your sex is generally referred to as female. Terms used to define sex include "male" and "female." The terms "sex" and "gender" are often used interchangeably, although they describe different yet related characteristics. The term "sex" as a verb can also be used to describe "the act" of "doing it," but for purposes of clarity, we can use terms such as "intercourse" or "sexual contact/behaviors" to describe this aspect of the term.

Gender can be defined as the behavioral, cultural, and psychological traits typically associated with one's sex. It is a term that really describes a set of social expectations about how one behaves in relation to what sex one is perceived to be.

Gender role or *sex role* is highly culturally and socially derived; it comes from the group, culture, or society one lives in. What is defined as being associated with a gender is determined by your group in a given period of time. For example, in white middle-class America in 1940, for a woman to wear trousers was considered *out* of her gender role. Today, it is normative. So, gender role can change, depending on the times, the culture, and who is in power. Terms that describe gender include "male," "female," and "transgender."

Gender identity is different from sexual orientation. It includes an internal sense of what sex a person is: his or her gender self-concept. Most people feel "at home" in their birth bodies. Some people feel strongly (for biological reasons) uncomfortable in their birth sex. Most of us think in terms of only two genders, but the more we are learning about gender and identity, the more we are beginning to understand that gender is complex and not just polarized. In fact, today there are some who would identify as *bigender*. Gender identity is not always derived from genital anatomy. Terms for individuals who experience gender identity dissonance include "transgender," "preoperative and postoperative transsexuals," "nonoperative transsexuals," and "gender queer." "Transitioning" is a term used to describe preoperative and postoperative transsexuals who are in the process of changing their bodies to be more congruent with their self-identified gender. "Transsexual" and "transgender" are terms that are often used interchangeably. Gender identity disorder, included in the *Diagnostic and Statistical Manual of Mental Disorders* (4th ed.), implies that most forms of transgender behavior are the results of gender identity dysphoria (or confliction with one's identity) and are symptoms of a clinically diagnosable psychiatric disorder. The accepted use of GID as a psychological disorder is controversial, and currently under consideration for removal or reevaluation as it is deemed harmful by many sexual health advocates.

A *transsexual* is a person who presents him- or herself and lives as the sex opposite his or her birth. Some transsexual individuals will transition physically to the opposite sex through hormonal and surgical procedures, although many cannot afford the multiple surgeries associated with physically transitioning and choose to live as the opposite sex through dress and/or hormonal treatments. Typically, a qualified sex therapist or psychologist will work with transsexuals so that they can make a healthy emotional adjustment. Living as the opposite sex for a minimum of one year is recommended in order for the person to begin to adjust to reactions from family members, work settings, and peers as well as their own feelings, although this form of therapy can be considered "gate-keeping" and a barrier to transition. Nonetheless, many individuals are able to transition and live comfortably in their new sex with adequate support and guidance.

Transgender is an umbrella term to describe the continuum of people whose gender identity and expression, to varying degrees, do not correspond with their genetic sex. As previously described, terms include "gender queer," "transsexual," "transgender," "bigender," and so on.

Gender expression has to do with the expression of gender and behaviors, including grooming, dress, and social interactions, which are associated with a particular gender in society. What is considered masculine in U.S. culture may not be in another country. Cultural norms can vary and change over time in terms of how gender expression is accepted. Expressing oneself in a masculine manner as a woman is viewed as "butch" in U.S. culture and is stereotypically associated with being lesbian, for example. "Androgyny" is a term that falls under gender expression, as do "masculine" and "feminine" as well as terms such as "butch/femme" for lesbians and "flaming," "queen," or "bear" for gay men (these examples are not exhaustive). Androgynous expression walks the line between genders; androgynous people are often mistaken for the opposite sex because of their nontraditional gender expression.

Gender role: is dependent on the culture one is born into or lives in. In U.S. culture, the gender role norm for boys and men is to be tough and independent, to hide emotion, and to engage in traditional careers, such as sports, business, and the trades; girls and women are expected to be vulnerable and emotional, caretakers, teachers, and nurses. When people step out of these roles, they often are treated with skepticism, disdain, and disapproval from those who ascribe to traditional roles.

An *ally:* is a person who supports and honors the struggles and issues and prejudice experienced by lesbian, gay, bisexual, and transgender (LGBT) people and who takes a stand against heterosexism, homophobia, biphobia, and transphobia by verbally defending the rights of LGBT individuals. Allies often are politically involved in the rights of LGBT people and actively work to support sexual diversity for all.

Sexual orientation describes one's attraction for, sexual desire for, and romantic attachments to others. For some people, they are attracted to people of the opposite sex; others are attracted to people of the same sex, and others may be attracted to people of either sex. We use the word "orientation" as more inclusive and appropriate than "preference" because the use of the word "preference" indicates a choice, which can in turn imply moral decision making. Although some LGBT individuals would say that their sexual orientation was a choice, many feel it is not a choice—that it is as inborn as in some other characteristics we have, like eye color or hair color. For civil purposes, it is easier and clearer to seek equal protection under the law for inborn characteristics than for something that can be perceived to be a choice, that is, a moral decision. Therefore, many in the community have advocated the concept of orientation over preference. Heterosexual, gay, straight, lesbian, bisexual, and homosexual are all sexual orientations. The term "queer" can be included under sexual orientation (or ally). Transgender or transsexual individuals, regardless of their gender identification, will self-define their sexual orientation according to their identified sex and romantic, sexual attraction (this gets really confusing for some people to wrap their minds around). It is best not to assume a person's sexual orientation; if we are confused and feel we need clarification, it is always better to ask a person so that we avoid making erroneous assumptions.

Sexual orientation has to do with who we are romantically attracted to. It's who our heart goes "pitter patter" for. Our palms sweat and heart races when the person we find attractive walks into the room. We may or may not act on those attractions, but it's a start on defining who we are. If we are attracted to people of the opposite sex, we are considered heterosexual or straight. If we are attracted to people of the same sex, we could identify as lesbian (female) or gay (male).

Within sexual orientation, there is a group of individuals we refer to as bisexual. They are attracted to people of both sexes and may have varying levels of attraction, behavior, and identity. There are many myths surrounding bisexuality, making it a more stigmatized identity than identifying as either lesbian or gay. Within the lesbian and gay culture, bisexuals are often viewed negatively, making it an identity that is marginalized by both straight and gay culture. Bisexual individuals often move between the worlds of "straight" and "gay," usually in monogamous relationships.

KINSEY SCALE

A well-known conceptualization of sexual orientation is the Kinsey Scale. Alfred Kinsey was one of the pioneering sexologists who studied human sexual behavior in the 1940s and 1950s. He and his researchers literally interviewed over 11,000 men and women about their sexual behavior and developed a scale to illustrate the fluidity in human sexual

KINSEY SCALE

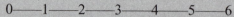

0. Exclusively heterosexual
1. Predominantly heterosexual, incidentally homosexual
2. Predominantly heterosexual but more than incidentally homosexual
3. Equally heterosexual and homosexual
4. Predominantly homosexual but more than incidentally heterosexual
5. Predominantly homosexual, incidentally heterosexual
6. Exclusively homosexual

behavior and attraction. Kinsey noted that, for many people, sexual behavior, thoughts, and feelings toward the same or opposite sex was not always consistent over time. Although the majority of men and women reported being exclusively heterosexual (or straight) and others reported exclusively homosexual behavior and attractions, many individuals disclosed behaviors or thoughts somewhere in between. The commonly cited statistic that 10 percent of the general population is homosexual refers to Kinsey's findings (Kinsey Institute, 2011). His research was criticized for not being a random sample and for the locations for some of the sampling itself. Other randomized and more recent studies (Michael, Gagnon, Laumann, & Kolata, 1994) cite a lower incidence, but within certain cultures, such as the drug culture, sexual minorities are even more prevalent.

ORIENTATION, BEHAVIOR, AND IDENTITY

Understanding the fluidity of sexual expression and the forms it can take across the life span can be difficult for some people to grasp. Often, we tend to assume that a person is of a certain sexual orientation by what we see. We see a man married to a woman and assume that he is heterosexual. If we see that same married man kissing another man with passion, we may think that he is gay but in the closet. He may well be, but he may also be bisexual. He may also have an arrangement with his spouse that allows him to act on his passion from time to time. In terms of his identity, that is personal to him and is what he chooses to call himself. He may call himself heterosexual but have attractions to other men.

The combinations of orientation, behavior, and identity may shift, depending on who he is with, or they may remain constant. The same married man may lose his spouse to death and become involved with another man. We may assume that he is gay because of the sex of his partner, but again this man may still have romantic attraction to women and identify as bisexual. But he moves on the scale or orientation depending on whom he is romantically involved with. In fact, if we aren't sure about someone's sexual orientation, we just need to ask how they define it for themselves.

Attraction and orientation can be viewed as the involuntary emotional and physical response of our bodies to others. Some individuals are attracted to muscular bodies or to wit and intelligence. Did you plan whom you were going to fall in love with, or did it just happen? Some people have varying levels of attraction to the same, opposite, or both genders. Attraction and orientation are not always static; sometimes it changes over time.

Behavior is what we do: how we express our feelings of attraction. Unlike attraction, a person's behavior involves making choices. We can be attracted to a person but choose not to act on how we feel. Because behavior is visible, it is often how others label our identity, which is not always congruent with how we might choose to label ourselves. A person's behavior alone does not define his or her sexual identity.

Sexual identity is the individual process of labeling and defining our sexual feelings and behaviors and is a personal process. We cannot accurately label another person, as each person must decide how he or she wishes to be identified. Some people are not familiar with certain terminology, may engage in same-sex behavior, but reject labels because of cultural or personal reasons. Others may identify strongly with an identity or just feel uncomfortable with their feelings and suppress them. It is important to make distinctions between these components in order to work effectively with sexual orientation and sexual behavior.

Issues around sexual identity shape our values, attitudes, and behaviors. The environment we grow up in affects how well we develop and adjust as sexual beings. Mainstream heterosexuals are typically supported for their sexual orientation by a heterosexist society. "Heterosexism" is a term that means that everything in life is supposed to be heterosexual, that everything deemed heterosexual is normal and acceptable in society, and that everything that is not heterosexual is out of the norm, unacceptable, and wrong. Societal institutions that support heterosexuality include marriage, religions, insurance benefits, and the ability to move through society openly expressing affection to a sexual partner without fear of reprisal or being harassed.

OPPRESSION AND STIGMA

Being LGBT carries social stigma. This stigmatization leads to many at-risk situations for this population, including homelessness, suicide, physical/verbal abuse, and chemical dependency (Grossman, 1997). The stress caused by this stigma has been offered as an explanation of why some gays, lesbians, and bisexuals use and abuse drugs and alcohol. This has been called "minority stress," which is the result of being a sexual minority in a predominantly antigay society (DiPlacido, 1998). Minority stress can cause some LGBT individuals to use and abuse alcohol and other drugs as a method of coping with societal discrimination and disapproval.

Psychologically, a person experiences an emotional toll that may manifest itself in the use of substances, depression, participation in high-risk behaviors due to personal neglect, or even suicide. And for the stigmatizing aspects of identity that a person cannot hide, the toll is equal or greater. Multiple stigmas typically exacerbate an already difficult existence. Having one or more social stigmas can be a daily onslaught of potential negative consequences, so having support, a positive self-image, and a healthy outlook is critical for sexual health. And being able to successfully manage this stress is crucial for survival in a heterosexist society.

There are many parallels between oppression and addiction representing, in part, the experience of being LGBT in our society. By not recognizing and understanding these similarities and knowing how to integrate positive/supportive experiences and opportunities into the treatment process, an agency sets these clients up for potential relapse, failure, and continued shame—the opposite goals of a recovery program. For the LGBT person, coming out to a predominantly heterosexual group can be threatening if not downright frightening.

Identity is about who we are and is like a tapestry—multilayered, beautiful, and complex all at the same time. Our identities should be a source of pride and joy in our lives, not ones that cause us to feel shame and disgust. An important lesson here for providers and clients is that we aren't born feeling ashamed of who we are. We learn our values and attitudes from others. We are influenced by the environment, family, genetics, school, peers, culture, and religion. To be told that part of who we are is defective or bad is not conducive to positive development. We can, however, learn how to transform negative messages into positive, healthy, life-affirming ones.

CONNECTIONS TO SUBSTANCE USE

Of 16 large-scale studies that focused on the prevalence of substance abuse in LGBT communities, there is general consensus that gay men and lesbians have greater substance abuse problems than non-LGBT men and women (Center for Substance Abuse Treatments [CSAT], 2001). This is due in part to the stigmatization of sexual minorities and subsequent oppression associated with being LGBT. Often, LGBT people use substances to cope with negative experiences as well as to socialize or feel able to be sexual.

Specific studies (Lewis, Saghir, & Robins, 1982; Morales & Graves, 1983) cite that approximately 30 percent of lesbians have an alcohol abuse problem; this is three times higher than the general population. Other studies show that gay men and women were heavier substance abusers than the general population (Hughes & Wilsnack, 1997; Skinner, 1994; Skinner & Otis, 1996). Prevalence of bisexuality and lesbian orientation in our current study with 215 women in treatment is just over 25 percent. From these studies, it is clear that substance abuse treatment is needed for LGBT persons and that providers need to know more about sexual orientation and sexuality issues in order to provide competent treatment services.

Research has shown that factors specific to the usage of alcohol and other drugs by LGBT persons include the lack of institutional supports, increased isolation due to lack of opportunities and fear of coming out, the bar scene (which for many is the only safe and acceptable place to socialize), and the homophobic attitudes and behavior of society, further contributing to the isolation and use of substance as a coping strategy (CSAT, 2001). Other literature (Hellman & Drescher, 2004) supports the provision of LGBT-specific groups and educational interventions as beneficial to the recovery process in the drug and alcohol and mental health fields.

INTERNALIZED HOMOPHOBIA

Internalized homophobia has also been identified as a factor affecting the higher levels of substance abuse among LGBT people. Internalized homophobia occurs when gays, lesbians, and bisexuals buy in to the negative attitudes projected at homosexuals, resulting in personal shame, guilt, and self-loathing. Anderson (2009) notes "the connection between sexual orientation and substance use disorders is often mediated by internalized homophobia . . . which can result in profound feelings of shame, depression, and self-hatred. Substances can then become part of a person's coping system" (p. 2). It is vital that LGBT clients have access to counselors who accept their sexual orientation. It is equally important that these clients have treatment that considers and is sensitive to their unique situation as sexual minorities. This can be the key on which their success in treatment turns.

ROLE OF COUNSELORS

There is a strong belief among substance abuse counselors that their clients are *only* in treatment to learn how to stop using. Attempts to integrate "special needs" groups are often met administratively and clinically with resistance, backed by claims that the client is just using his or her sexual orientation as an excuse to isolate him- or herself from recovery efforts within a generic group setting. This mentality misses the point of cultural isolation due to clients "keeping secrets" for fear of being ostracized, ridiculed, shamed, and/or not being supported in therapy if they choose to "come out" to their generic groups, or, even worse, negative feedback is supported or encouraged by the counselor. We need to provide support, realizing that our attitudes can retraumatize LGBT clients who have previously experienced trauma around their sexual and gender orientation.

Because each client brings his or her own unique history and background into treatment, furthering our understanding of individuals different from ourselves helps ensure that clients are treated with respect while improving the likelihood of effective substance abuse treatment interventions. A substance abuse treatment provider who is knowledgeable about the unique needs of LGBT clients can enhance treatment. A provider who understands and is sensitive to the issues surrounding sexual and gender identity, homophobia, and heterosexism can help LGBT clients feel comfortable and safe while they confront their substance abuse and start their journey of recovery (CSAT, 2001).

Shame is a powerful force and is a huge issue for substance abusers, one that will contribute to relapse and continued self-harm if not arrested and transformed. Sexual identity can be one of the biggest sources of shame for people, one that has no place in drug and alcohol treatment. A treatment agency that does not affirm sexuality and respect the right to love whom we are attracted to promotes an environment that embraces inequality, prejudice, hate, and discrimination.

CLIENT EXPERIENCES

We all grew up in the same world regardless of our sexual and gender orientation. That means that we all heard the same messages about what it meant to be gay, including witnessing the name-calling, stereotyping, and harassment. Some of those messages included being told that gays were morally corrupt, deviant, child molesters, sinners, or worse. If we grew up knowing that we were gay or lesbian, many of us internalized the messages, learning how to hate ourselves for being LGBT or experiencing discomfort for having same-sex attractions. *Being* LGBT is not a choice; whether we choose to act on it is the only choice involved.

One client (age 24) shared about messages they learned growing up:

> Um, my parents didn't necessarily say, don't have sex until marriage, they were more, my mom was more realistic, like be safe if you're going to, but growing up I had an uncle, who is gay and my parents were very like, that's not okay, like whatsoever and they weren't really religious, but if you were gay you were going to hell. But the uncle is still part of our family, they would say "that's disgusting and immoral and it's a choice and I don't know why anyone would choose that" so growing up, what I started realizing was that I was attracted to girls and I was kind of uncomfortable with that and it's still hard for me cuz in the last six months, my own spirituality has really been growing and I identify myself as a Christian now, but I still, I don't, I have a hard time, I don't believe that that, that its okay that I'm bisexual. I believe that, but it's still hard for me, I still struggle with that sometimes cuz it was so in ground in my brain.

Unfortunately, many LGBT individuals decide to hide who they are from others for fear of societal reprisal. Others come to a point where they cannot or do not want to hide and choose to "come out" to other people. Levels of coming out include personal (to oneself), interpersonal (to another), social (to a group of friends or acquaintances), or public (in a forum in that a larger group of strangers is informed, such as at seminars or on radio or television). If a client is using, in part, to not deal with their sexual orientation, then it will need to be part of their treatment plan in order to help prevent relapse associated with the feelings of fear and/or self-loathing.

Coming out is a joyful and liberating experience, or it can be one of the most devastating events a person goes through. Families have ostracized their LGBT children, kicked them out of the home, disowned them, and literally physically assaulted them. A negative response to a coming-out experience can influence a person's desire to cover up emotional pain through the use of drugs or alcohol. Consequences of coming out in the form of loss of familial support or relationships can further damage the psyche and contribute to a downward spiral of depression or substance use. Take, for example, this client's experiences:

> Yea, I tried for a really long time to say you know what, I can do this, but I, I would walk into a bar and all of the people that before you

know [before coming out] and they'd be like hey Kandy [not a real name], what's goin on and all of these acquaintances, all of these fake friends that you just love to talk to when your drinking. After I came out I'd walk into a bar and everybody would like just look at me. You know, turn their heads and psst psst psst, and finally somebody would say, "O hi." I think to myself, you gotta be fucking kidding me. And that took my self-esteem into, into, you know, I didn't have any. And I isolated. My girlfriend and I completely isolated.

Or, coming out to her coworkers and family:

I wound up dating my boss. One of my best friends worked with me and this um, was her boss as well and had to start telling my friends, I had to tell them what was going on, somebody was gonna find out. And I uh, decided to come out and let them know and uh, it was very traumatic. They all started crying, you know. Some of them were very angry and pissed. When I went to my mother her face you know, shriveled up like this you know, this distorted devilish prune and she spit on me [laughs] you know and I was like what the hell is this? The one time I actually decide to open up to you, maybe start a new relationship here, and this is what I get. You want to get to know me, you've always said I don't talk to you I don't whatever, and here you go.

Coming out can also create stress with regard to peer rejection, abandonment, and loss of housing or employment. Although there are more places that include sexual orientation as an area of equal rights, most states and places of employment do not protect against discrimination from sexual or gender orientation. Being supported in coming out, knowing who to come out to, why or why not to come out, and how to come out are areas that may need to be addressed in helping someone deal with their substance use. If the person has been self-medicating in order to deal with being LGBT, then being clean and sober and having to navigate coming out and/or internalized homophobia will be critical to a successful recovery.

OTHER LINKS TO SUBSTANCE USE

Prostitution and homelessness contribute to LGBT substance use and abuse. When young people are kicked out of the home, they may have to turn to illegal acts or prostitution to support themselves, and these homeless youth are vulnerable to sexual exploitation. Youth who are LGBT have the highest risk of suicide among adolescents, and it is unfortunate that they feel there is no way out of a temporarily painful situation. Again, the thread of shame over being put out of the home, disowned, abandoned, told they are worthless, or having to trade sex for money, drugs, or a place to stay, coupled with an uncertain future, are factors that can pave the way for subsequent addiction, sexual risk, or death from violence or overdose.

There is an increased incidence of substance abuse among this population because of cultural learning that states that LGBT persons rely heavily on bars as a culturally prescribed setting for social interaction or as a resource for responding to stress (McKirnan & Peterson, 1989). Within the LGBT community, gay bars have historically served in the critical capacity of providing refuge from homophobia and stigmatization: the one definitive place where one can be oneself and be accepted. Drugs and alcohol figure prominently within many LGBT social settings (such as nightclubs, pride events, and circuit parties). The availability/accessibility of substances, in addition to cultural norms that are accepting of substance use, are identified risk factors for substance abuse. Other links to substance use with regard to sexual identity include the use of specific drugs with regard to sexual enhancement (methamphetamines and gay men), cocaine, alcohol expectancies, and so on.

CLIENT HOMEWORK

A suggested homework assignment for LGBT clients would be to ask them to find a local newspaper or website for LGBT people and to make a list of all the social activities that are listed. They should make a note of which ones are not centered on the bar scene and pick out a couple that they might be willing to explore in terms of a sober social environment. Being able to explore options and alternatives to trigger situations can help LGBT clients find healthier methods for building sober social networks.

CREATING THE CONTEXT FOR TREATMENT

From the outset, it is essential that clients know that the program/agency is LGBT affirming. The best-case scenario does not single out individual clients who are assumed to be LGBT; rather, it makes this affirmation as a statement of general fact. As counselors, we should remember that such assumptions cannot and should not be made. Sexual orientation and sexual identity are different: clients may present a public persona that is contrary to his or her sexual orientation. We also may not know the stage at which clients are in their coming-out process.

Counselors should be aware of the ways in which acceptance of sexual orientation is reflected. An overall comfort with discussion(s) of sexual orientation is one way that this is accomplished. Use of inclusive language is another key element, as is a nonjudgmental attitude. Unspoken cues, such as body language, send significant messages of acceptance and affirmation. In group settings, ground rules that prohibit name-calling, jokes, and bias offers reassurance to LGBT members that they are in a safe environment.

SELF-ASSESSMENT AND COUNTERTRANSFERENCE

Counselors should be very aware of how their own ambivalent or negative attitudes affect LGBT clients. A deep, honest look at one's own feelings about homosexuality and bisexuality is an absolute must. It has been asserted that client perceptions of the therapeutic relationship factors account for 30 percent of successful outcome (Asay & Lambert, 1999). The client's perceptions of the therapeutic alliance have been estimated to account for 54 percent of therapeutic gains (Wampold, 2001). The therapeutic alliance is critical—we are, after all, in partnership with the client in order to effect change in the client's behavior/life. If we are harboring antigay sentiments, we will undoubtedly damage the relational bond that is vital for successful treatment outcomes.

Substance abuse counselors have considerable power and influence over the recovery process of clients; therefore, their attitudes may significantly affect clients' chances of recovery. The role of cultural competence has increased significantly over the past decade, yet many individuals think about race and ethnicity when they consider diversity issues. It is important for counselors to incorporate other forms of diversity in their treatment approaches in order to be aware of and sensitive to a variety of cultures, including gender and sexual orientation. Before we begin to work with sexual orientation and gender identity issues, it is helpful to start with ourselves. Completing a self-assessment can help us identify personal attitudes and bias. For example, if our religious upbringing impacted how we feel about homosexuality, we may hold negative attitudes toward sexual orientations other than straight; this can transfer to the therapeutic setting. Counselors will be on their way to being well rounded once they have done a personal assessment and taken steps to identify any bias, acquired further training, and know what their limitations are, if any.

ASSESSING ATTITUDES TOWARD HOMOSEXUALITY

Dorothy Riddle (1985) developed a scale that measures personal bias and attitudes toward homosexuality. This tool can aid individuals in assessing their attitudes toward homosexuality. Attitudes can range from repulsed to nurturing, and subcategories of each are further explored in the scale. Taking an honest appraisal of our biases requires rigorous honesty. Let's face it: it's not easy to admit we have shortcomings. I have done this work for years and do not identify as straight, yet my own internal feelings and bias range on a continuum. Moving forward on the continuum is the goal. Being honest requires courage and the ability to look at how we internalize societal messages. What was learned *can* be unlearned if we are willing to work on it. As human service professionals, we have an obligation to serve our clients with dignity and respect.

COMING-OUT AND SELF-DISCLOSURE

Once a self-assessment has been done, the next steps would include understanding the coming-out process, stages of sexual identity development, and learning how to incorporate these tools in a counseling environment. There are numerous levels that someone can come out on; these are indicated on pages 52–54. "Coming out" is a term used to describe when individuals acknowledge to themselves or another person that they are LGBT or that they are even questioning their identities.

Self-disclosure can be one of the greatest challenges facing counselors who work with LGBT clients. Many members of the LGBT community have faced the discrimination and outright rejection that comes with homophobia. LGBT persons have experienced or witnessed verbal harassment, discrimination in employment/housing, estrangement from family and friends, and even assault. It is important to recognize that this can occur within the broader society, within the family unit, and within the client in the event that they are experiencing internalized homophobia.

Some clients have experienced this discrimination and disapproval within the very service institutions that they have turned to for assistance: shelters, social service agencies, and substance abuse treatment centers. These negative experiences related to disclosure of their sexual orientation can have a lasting impact on our clients, making subsequent disclosures less likely and difficult to attain. A client's hesitancy to come out should be understood as the protective mechanism that it is for the client's psychological and, in some cases, physical well-being.

ATTITUDE TOWARD DIFFERENCE SURVEY: THE RIDDLE SCALE

Put a check next to each statement with which you agree. Bracket the two or three consecutive statements that reflect your current range of thinking about lesbian, gay, bisexual, and transgendered (LGBT) people.

☐   1. Homosexuality is unnatural and immoral. LGBT people are emotionally or psychologically ill.
☐   2. LGBT people should participate in reparative therapy or any other treatment available to help them change their sexual orientation.
☐   3. We should have compassion for LGBT people. They can't be blamed for how they were born.
☐   4. LGBT people didn't choose to be the way they are. If they could somehow become heterosexual, they would surely do so.
☐   5. Homosexuality is a phase that many people go through and most grow out of.
☐   6. LGBT people need our support and guidance as they wrestle with the many difficult issues associated with their lifestyle.
☐   7. I have no problem with LGBT people, but see no need for them to flaunt their sexual orientation publicly.
☐   8. What LGBT people do in the privacy of their own bedroom is their business.
☐   9. LGBT people deserve the same rights and privileges as everybody else.
☐ 10. Homophobia is wrong. Society needs to take a stand against anti-LGBT bias.
☐ 11. It takes strength and courage for LGBT people to be themselves in today's world.
☐ 12. It is important for me to examine my own attitudes so that I can actively support the struggle for equality that LGBT people have undertaken.
☐ 13. There is great value in our human diversity. LGBT people are an important part of that diversity.
☐ 14. It is important for me to stand up to those who demonstrate homophobic attitudes.
☐ 15. LGBT people are an indispensable part of our society. They have contributed much to our world and there is much to be learned from their experiences.

☐ 16. I would be proud to be part of an LGBT organization, and to
openly advocate for the full and equal inclusion of LGBT
people at all levels of our society.

ATTITUDES TOWARD DIFFERENCE SURVEY SCORING GUIDE

Find the numbers below that correspond to the bracketed range on
your survey. Read the attitude and characteristics that encompass
this range. According to the Attitudes toward Difference Scale
developed by psychologist Dorothy Riddle, this is where you stand
with regard to LGBT people.

RANGE ATTITUDE CHARACTERISTICS

1–2	Repulsion	LGBT people are strange, sick, crazy and aversive.
3–4	Pity	LGBT people are somehow born that way and it is pitiful.
5–6	Tolerance	Life for LGBT people is hard; anti-gay attitudes just make things worse.
7–8	Acceptance	Homosexuality is a fact of life that should neither be punished nor celebrated.
9–10	Support	The rights of LGBT people should be protected and safeguarded.
11–12	Admiration	Being LGBT in our society takes strength.
13–14	Appreciation	There is value in diversity. Homophobic attitudes should be confronted.
15–16	Nurturance	LGBT people are an indispensable part of society.

Adapted from Riddle (1985).

YOUR RATING

1–4 Your personal feelings may be preventing you from accepting
and respecting LGBT people.

5–8 You are somewhat accepting, but may not be willing to actively
work against anti-LGBT bias.

9–12 You are willing to provide support and work toward equal rights
for LGBT people.

13–16 You are able to fully embrace LGBT people as equal and
valuable members of the community.

FOOD FOR THOUGHT
- ❑ Are your attitudes toward LGBT people based upon experience or preconceptions?
- ❑ Are you as accepting of LGBT people as you are of people from different racial, ethnic or religious backgrounds? Why or why not?
- ❑ Have you ever had an LGBT friend? How might your attitudes help or hinder you from being an ally for LGBT people?
- ❑ What can you do educate yourself about LGBT issues and improve your attitude with regard to LGBT people?

Adapted from GLSEN, 2002.

Coming out is a complex and ongoing process that must be respected by substance abuse counselors if we are to provide a safe, affirming atmosphere conducive to reparative change for our LGBT clients. It is critical, however, that coming out (at least to those who are of significance to the client) be explored in the treatment setting. Many treatment facilities have no LGBT-identified staff members. There is a high probability that LGBT clients will experience substance abuse counseling with counselors who have had no training on providing LGBT-specific substance abuse treatment. Some studies have revealed that 50 percent of substance abuse counselors have received no training at all about LGBT issues in substance abuse counseling (Eliason, 2000). LGBT clients face unique challenges in recovery. As a result, treatment plans should reflect a cognizance of this and be tailored to meet the needs of this segment of the substance-abusing population.

In the preaware stage, a person is not aware of his or her sexual orientation as being anything except heterosexual. This stage is akin to being precontemplative in the stages of change model. The person may also have had some inklings of being different in this stage but is denying to him- or herself or others that it has nothing to do with his or her sexual orientation.

COMING-OUT CONTINUUM OF EXPERIENCE

>............>...........>...........>.........>........>........>
   Preaware   Personal Interpersonal   Social   Public

The personal stage of coming out is when individuals admit to themselves that they are or might be LGBT. They may or may not choose to tell another person and may also keep this information to themselves. There is no prescribed time limit on this or other stages. It can happen as a child, adolescent, young adult, or older adult. Whether a person decides to come out is contingent on myriad factors.

In the interpersonal stage, individuals tell other people that they are or might be LGBT. There are no rules on who individuals decide to tell. It is usually someone they feel will not betray their confidence. In the event the experience is a negative one, they may go back "into the closet," choose to not tell other people, or continue to seek support. Often, when teens come out and it starts to become common knowledge among their peers in a school setting, teasing, bullying, and violent behaviors can ensue. Even though there is more awareness and support for LGBT youth in schools and society, the negative behaviors from others continue to be problematic and often quite disturbing. Supporting and connecting teens (or any persons) who are coming out to others is critical to personal acceptance of a healthy sexual identity development.

Social coming out pertains to the process of the LGBT person developing a group of friends, typically in loose social settings. For some LGBT individuals, this includes the bar scene, where they may have gone in order to meet other people. Online forums are common and can be a safe place (alcohol and drug free) to meet other people, discuss concerns around coming out, and develop a social network. An online forum can be particularly helpful for people who live in rural areas, where coming out and meeting others could be dangerous.

Coming out on a public level happens when LGBT people typically do advocacy work, and are speaking out at community meetings, conferences, television and news, and so on. Examples of publicly known LGBT people are Ellen Degeneres, Chaz Bono, Elton John, and k.d. lang. When individuals "out" themselves in any public forum, they are taking a risk as well as advocating for those who cannot. Public discussion of sexual and gender orientation can be viewed as a positive way to educate others, normalize identity issues, and dispel harmful myths about what it is like to be LGBT.

RECOGNITION OF THE POIGNANCY OF THE COMING-OUT EVENT/PROCESS

Counselors should operate with the knowledge that coming out is a pivotal life moment for their LGBT clients. This can refer to the knowledge/realization of one's same-sex attraction and/or the revelation of one's sexual orientation to others. The initial realization of same-sex attraction can be a source of internal turmoil for some clients—an event with which they may still be grappling. For others, this personal acknowledgment was a positive, relief-inducing moment. In either case, counselors should not overlook or ignore the coming-out event as significant for our LGBT clients and should reflect genuine interest in discussing and exploring this subject in treatment.

STIGMA MANAGEMENT

Since coming out is an ongoing process that is reinitiated every time a client is in a new situation or meets new people, we should be aware as counselors that our clients are never "done" with coming out and its social consequences. We also need to make sure we do not force clients to come-out in situations that may be harmful to their psychological well-being. Asking clients to come-out to family members who may reject them, or peers who may treat them abusively is asking them to risk rejection and potential relapse. This form of ongoing "stigma management," or developing the internal sense of knowing who it is safe to come-out to, where and why, is a critical piece of the treatment and recovery process.

As practitioners in the substance abuse field become more cognizant of the importance of multiculturalism in the application of our practice, we cannot overlook LGBT substance abusers and their individualized needs. This, therefore, requires a commitment of education, introspection, and training on the part of counselors to ensure that we are imparting the best care that we can in a manner that does not retraumatize our clients. Unlike racial minorities (whose identities, for the most part, are visibly seen), sexual minorities are not so readily identified. With this potential for anonymity, we can never be completely sure whether we are addressing an LGBT client. We should just assume that we are. If there is the perception that counselors have to "go the extra mile" regarding LGBT clients, perhaps that is true.

SEXUAL IDENTITY DEVELOPMENT

Vivian Cass, an Australian psychologist, developed a model of sexual identity development that can be helpful in staging oneself in the process of self-acceptance. Her stages illustrate various developmental tasks that need to happen in order for a person to move forward in self-acceptance of a healthy sexual identity (as well as recovery). Being able to stage clients in their sexual identity development can help counselors determine how to best support them in this process.

CASS'S MODEL OF LESBIAN AND GAY IDENTITY DEVELOPMENT

(adapted to include bisexual, transgender, and recovery processes)

Stage I: Identity Confusion
Occurs when a person begins to realize that he or she may relate to and/or identify themselves with being LGBT; a process of *personalizing the identity*.
Tasks: Exploration and increasing awareness
Feelings: Anxiety, confusion
Defenses: Denial
Recovery: Having a confidential support person

Stage II: Identity Comparison
Occurs when a person *accepts the possibility that he or she might be LGBT*.
Tasks: Exploration of implications; encountering others like oneself
Feelings: Anxiety, excitement
Defenses: Bargaining and rationalizing
Recovery: Meeting LGBT people in recovery

Stage III: Identity Tolerance
Occurs when a person comes to *accept the probability that he or she is LGBT*.
Tasks: Recognizing social and emotional needs as an LGBT person
Feelings: Anger, excitement
Defenses: Reactivity
Recovery: How to be LGBT and stay sober

Stage IV: Identity Acceptance
Occurs when a person *fully accepts rather than tolerates themselves as LGBT*.
Tasks: Development of community and acculturation
Feelings: Rage and sadness
Defenses: Hostility toward straight culture
Recovery: LGBT community building

Stage V: Identity Pride
Occurs when the person *immerses themselves in LGBT community and culture to totally live out the identity.*
Tasks: Full experience of being LGBT, confronting internalized homophobia
Feelings: Excitement and focused anger
Defenses: Arrogant pride and rejection of straight culture as the norm
Recovery: Sexuality, identity and recovery

Stage VI: Identity Synthesis
Occurs when a person develops a *fully internalized and integrated LGBT identity and experiences themselves as whole when interacting with everyone across all environments.*
Tasks: Coming out as fully as possible; intimate LGBT relationship; self-actualization as LGBT
Feelings: Excitement and happiness
Defenses: Minimal
Recovery: Maintenance

Adapted from New York State Office of Alcohol and Substance Abuse Services.

Cass's (1979) six-stage theory developed from a psychosocial perspective (Levine, 1997) and is based on interpersonal congruency theory (Cox & Gallois, 1996). Motivation for development is viewed as the need to reduce the incongruence that each stage creates interpersonally and in reference to society (Cox & Gallois, 1996). Individuals either work through each stage or undergo identity foreclosure, terminating forward movement in the homosexual identity formation process (Cass, 1984).

The first stage of Cass's theory is identity confusion. The onset of this stage is characterized by the first conscious awareness that homosexuality has relevance to oneself in terms of one's behavior, thoughts, or feelings. During this stage, one realizes that one's behavior or feelings could be defined as homosexual (Cox & Gallois, 1996), which raises the question of whether one is gay, lesbian, or bisexual. Inner turmoil and feelings of personal alienation characterize this stage (Cass, 1979). Unless identity foreclosure occurs, the confused person naturally moves into the second stage: identity comparison.

The identity comparison stage is marked by a tentative commitment to the homosexual self. The main task of this stage is to handle the social alienation that results as one becomes increasingly aware of the differences between oneself and others (Cass, 1979). There are several ways people typically handle social alienation. Some respond positively to the notion that they are different and thus become further inclined to accept their identity, while others realize that they are gay, lesbian, or bisexual and therefore different but find that undesirable and therefore seek to change their perception of their behavior as being gay, lesbian, or bisexual. People who fall into this latter category often consider a sexual relationship they may be involved in as a special case or believe that they could act heterosexual if they chose to do so. They may convince themselves that this is a temporary identity, or they may blame someone else so as to maintain their personal innocence (Cass, 1979). Others may recognize they are gay but seek to change their behaviors because of the perceived undesirability of being gay (Cass, 1979). The final response to the incongruence of stage 2 is to attempt to change one's perception of oneself as being gay, lesbian, or bisexual as well as discontinue any behaviors that are considered homosexual. If the client succeeds in making these changes, identity foreclosure occurs and no further progress is made in the homosexual identity formation progress. If it is unsuccessful, there is usually a dangerous amount of self-hatred and increased risk of self-harm (Cass, 1979).

If stage 2 is handled healthily, then one moves from "I might be gay" to "I probably am gay" and thus into stage 3: identity tolerance (Cass, 1979). The sense of alienation is heightened, and other sexual minorities are sought out to alleviate feelings of aloneness (Cox & Gallois, 1996). The critical factor in this stage is the emotional quality of the contact with other gay, lesbian, or bisexual people (Cass, 1979). If one sees one's homosexual self-image as undesirable, a positive contact in this stage can lead to a reevaluation of the negative perception. If the experience is a negative one, it increases one's negative self-concept. If identity foreclosure does not occur, one is led to greater commitment to their gay, lesbian, or bisexual identity.

Stage 4, identity acceptance, is characterized by increased contact with other gay, lesbian, or bisexual people and a sense of feeling normal (Sophie, 1986). Other sexual minorities are viewed more positively, and the gay subculture becomes increasingly important in one's life. The incongruence between how one views oneself and how one thinks others see one is heightened, creating a natural move into stage 5.

Stage 5, identity pride, is characterized by a nearly complete acceptance of one's gay, lesbian, or bisexual self, coupled with an acute awareness of the rejection of gays, lesbians, or bisexuals by society (Cass, 1979). The world is often seen as divided into two camps: heterosexual and homosexual. One's commitment to the homosexual group, or sense of identity, is very strong. This often leads to activism and purposeful confrontation with the establishment (Cass, 1979). In this stage, one's gay, lesbian, or bisexual identity is the primary identity, superseding all other aspects of one's life. The disclosing of one's sexuality to others is likely to increase; how others' responses are perceived has a great impact on whether development continues. When disclosing of a minority sexual orientation results in an unexpected positive response on the part of a heterosexual, the individual recognized the inconsistency of his or her thoughts and moves naturally into the final stage of development.

The last stage, identity synthesis, is reached when the sexual minority individual is able to integrate one's homosexual self with other important aspects of one's identity. Being gay, lesbian, or bisexual is no longer seen as one's sole identity but rather as a part (though an important one) of the whole picture of who one is (Cass, 1979). There is increased contact with supportive heterosexuals, and one's personal and public sexual identities become more unified.

TREATMENT CONSIDERATIONS

Considering the Kinsey scale, the coming-out process, and the Cass model, what are some ways you might be able to utilize these tools in a clinical setting? How might you determine "where your client is at" in terms of sexual orientation, coming out, or their sexual identity development? How might you best support them in their process of recovery with regard to these stage models? Remember, pushing a client where they are not ready to go themselves can set up resistance or even risk for relapse. We need to be able to make sure a client is okay with the process, is willing and able to move forward, and has the skills to cope with any associated stressors of the next phase of coming out and so on.

Attending trainings on sexual orientation that are geared toward values clarification and attitude reassessment are recommended. Proper screening, use of language, referral tools, and agency assessment are important considerations for developing and fostering a healthy environment for treating the LGBT substance abuser.

LGBT clients need special consideration of their sexual and gender orientation in order to recover from addiction and reduce the likelihood

ASSESSMENT AND INTERVENTION CHECKLIST

1. Gathering intake information to provide opportunities for coming out and being genuine:
   • Are you in a committed relationship with a man or woman, and for how long?
   • LGBT affirmative literature on display in counselor's office
2. Taking a family history that is inclusive of alternative families and other critical social networks; determining how ostracized one may be within the family unit for being LGBT:
   • Is your family supportive of you?
   • Who do you consider as part of your "family" network (explore alternative families)?
3. Taking a psych and treatment history that acknowledges when clients have been psychopathologized for being LGBT and/or subsequently mistreated in previous treatment:
   • Were you ever pushed into therapy or treatment because you were LGBT?
   • How LGBT affirmative or insensitive were your former treatment experiences/last counselor?
4. Exploring sexuality in a supportive, nonconfrontative manner:
   • How would you describe your romantic and/or sexual orientation?

LGBT SUPPORTIVE ENVIRONMENT ASSESSMENT

Evaluate your current level of support. Consider each statement and write Yes for those that are true and No for those that are not.

_____ My agency has LGBT support groups.
_____ My agency has an identified counselor for LGBT issues.
_____ Contributions of LGBT person's are acknowledged and shared in my agency's work.
_____ My agency's affirmative action statement for staff and clients includes sexual orientation and gender identity/or gender expression.

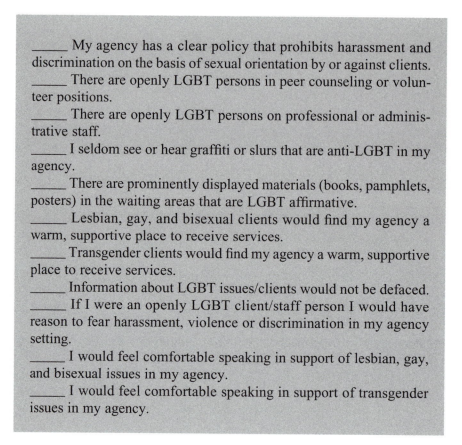

_____ My agency has a clear policy that prohibits harassment and discrimination on the basis of sexual orientation by or against clients.

_____ There are openly LGBT persons in peer counseling or volunteer positions.

_____ There are openly LGBT persons on professional or administrative staff.

_____ I seldom see or hear graffiti or slurs that are anti-LGBT in my agency.

_____ There are prominently displayed materials (books, pamphlets, posters) in the waiting areas that are LGBT affirmative.

_____ Lesbian, gay, and bisexual clients would find my agency a warm, supportive place to receive services.

_____ Transgender clients would find my agency a warm, supportive place to receive services.

_____ Information about LGBT issues/clients would not be defaced.

_____ If I were an openly LGBT client/staff person I would have reason to fear harassment, violence or discrimination in my agency setting.

_____ I would feel comfortable speaking in support of lesbian, gay, and bisexual issues in my agency.

_____ I would feel comfortable speaking in support of transgender issues in my agency.

of relapse. Counselors need training and support in order to facilitate this process. Client treatment groups or support groups will give LGBT clients a safe place to discuss their sexuality issues. Ignoring sexuality issues of LGBT persons ignores an integral part of their core being, therefore contributing to a deeper negative self-image and further harming them. Supporting sexuality issues of LGBT persons in treatment will assist them in developing (perhaps for the first time) a positive self-concept of themselves and a legitimate part of society.

RESOURCES ON SEXUAL ORIENTATION AND GENDER IDENTITY

Books and Manuals

Anderson, S. C. (2009). *Substance use disorders in lesbian, gay, bisexual and transgender clients: Assessment and treatment*. New York: Columbia University Press.

Brill, S., & Pepper, R. (2008). *The transgender child: A handbook for families and professionals.* Berkeley, CA: Cleis Press.

Kaufman, G., & Raphael, L. (1996). *Coming out of shame: Transforming gay and lesbian lives.* New York: Bantam Doubleday Dell Publishing Group.

Substance Abuse and Mental Health Services Administration. (2001). *A provider's introduction to substance abuse treatment for lesbian, gay, bisexual, and transgender individuals.* http://store.samhsa.gov/product/A-Provider-s-Introduction-to-Substance-Abuse-Treatment-for-Lesbian-Gay-Bisexual-and-Transgender-Individuals/SMA09-4104.

Online Resources

CenterLink. Local, State and National LGBT Organizations and Groups. http://www.lgbtcenters.org/localstatenational-groups.aspx.

GLBTT Health: Get It On. http://www.getiton.ca/index.php.

International Lesbian, Gay, Bisexual, Trans and Intersex Association. http://ilga.org/ilga/en/index.html.

National Association of Lesbian, Gay, Bisexual and Transgender Addiction Professionals and Their Allies: LGBT resources. http://www.nalgap.org/resources.htm.

Substance Abuse Treatment Resources for the GLBT Community. http://www.chestnut.org/li/apss/Common/Multicultural/GLTBQ_Resources.pdf.

FOUR

The "Blue-Light" Special

Whoever called it necking was a poor judge of anatomy.

—Groucho Marx

Just the facts, ma'am. What did you learn about sexuality growing up from your school? Chances are, if you learned anything at all about sex, it was about the facts, the plumbing, how things work. Many of us did not even learn that much, depending on what kind of school we went to. More of us learned about sex from our friends, and we know how sketchy that type of learning can be. Some sexologists fondly refer to this spoke of the wheel as the "blue-light" special, those of us who are old enough to remember that blue light flashing at K-mart, advertising the special of the hour. That same blue light flashes in some schools all over America—just the facts kids!

This chapter is not all about the facts; in fact, little about the facts is presented in terms of anatomy and physiology. This chapter discusses some facts in terms of human sexual development, issues that may go awry or impact substance use and vice versa, and we will learn about how to incorporate values clarification activities into sexual health programming and address bias in ourselves and our clients. Some excellent resources are provided at the end of the chapter so that you can brush up on the facts if you need to. We will discuss how we can effectively teach the facts and other key learning factors that will increase your ability to provide effective treatment learning environments and counseling tips. Becoming an effective sexual health educator does not come from just reading a book or taking a class. Skill develops over time with practice as well as by reading, attending seminars, and being open to a particular way of thinking. My hope is that this chapter will help move you gently in that direction.

Many schools teach from an abstinence base, and some of them provide inaccurate information regarding condoms as a fear tactic to scare kids away from having sex, but all this does is to create unprepared teenagers who have no idea what would prevent disease or pregnancy other than not "doing it." And for adolescents who are already sexually active, this leaves them unprepared for how to have healthy sexual relationships or how to stay safe from unwanted consequences associated with sexual activity. Comprehensive sexuality programs teach about sexuality from K–12 incorporating age-appropriate material in the curriculum. Many schools merely teach a few class sessions about anatomy and disease as part of a larger health class at specific grade levels. This approach leaves much to be desired in terms of how to assist youth in learning to negotiate relationships, safer sex, abuse, understanding intimacy and more.

SEXUAL DEVELOPMENT

Developmentally, there are sexual milestones that occur in stages as we grow and age. From birth to puberty, children will grow physically, cognitively, and emotionally. Although there is a great deal of sexual information and messages that can be taught during this time, conversations in school settings and at home are often absent. Children should be learning about how to correctly identify body parts (including sexual ones), know that people can have children only after they reach puberty, that their bodies will change as they grow older, that men and women have reproductive organs that can allow them to have a child, that when a woman is pregnant the baby grows inside her body in the uterus (not her stomach), that not all men and women want to have children, and that some people who cannot have children can adopt them. If parents have adequately prepared their children for puberty, the embarrassment, shame, and trauma that can accompany changes in the body through first menarche and nocturnal emissions will be minimized.

This list is certainly not exhaustive, and the subsequent sections also provide partial lists of relevant information related to sexual development. When children have sexuality questions, age-appropriate answers should be provided to correctly address them. Parents have a responsibility to engage in frank discussions around sexual issues in order to keep the lines of communication open. Typically, the younger the child, the less complicated answering questions will be. Often parents are not sure how detailed the information should be and end up avoiding discussions because of their lack of knowledge or embarrassment. An excellent resource for helping parents talk about healthy sexuality with their children is Advocates for Youth (http://www.advocatesforyouth.org).

Puberty

Once puberty begins, a number of changes will occur, including production of testosterone in males and estrogen/progesterone in females. In girls, physical changes include the development of breasts, increase in vaginal lubrication, ovulation, and menstruation and in boys darkening of the scrotum, deepening of the voice, sperm production, and more frequent erections and wet dreams. Youth are often anxious about pubertal changes and may be shy about asking questions of caregivers. They typically begin to feel conscious of their sexual selves and sexual expression and may have questions about what is normal sexual behavior, such as masturbation.

As youth move through adolescence, they will begin to express themselves sexually, which may or may not include sexual intercourse, and they should know about pregnancy and sexually transmitted infections and how to avoid them and should know about the possible consequences of intercourse. Some youth will be late developers, and others may experience changes earlier; this is normal and individual. Of course, being on one end of the spectrum or the other can create an environment of difference and may result in teasing and harassment from peers. Being ostracized for differences can be problematic if youth do not have a healthy support system. Youth should be learning about what constitutes healthy and unhealthy relationships and that they have the capacity to form loving, intimate relationships with other people. Loving, intimate relationships do not necessarily include sexual activity, as we define intimacy as the ability to be vulnerable and show affection to another human being and have that affection returned. We can have a loving, intimate relationship with our family of origin (nonsexual of course). A firm sense of their sexual orientation should be established, and teens should be aware that they are sexual beings and be able to understand the consequences of being sexual, preferably in a realistic, nonscary manner.

Early Sexual Messages

Having the capacity to discuss these changes and how they affect development and relationships is critical. Youth who receive shaming and humiliating messages about their budding sexuality will begin to develop a poor self-image that can be a risk factor for substance use. Parents who are uncomfortable discussing sexual development may ignore children's request for information or, even worse, joke and embarrass their child in order to avoid any conversations. The effects of being shamed and embarrassed can be detrimental for development and inadvertently teach youth that sexuality is bad and embarrassing and can foster discomfort in discussing sexual matters throughout adolescence and early adulthood. This type of environment can be a risk factor for sexual risk-taking behaviors, including unprotected sex, inappropriate sexual expression toward others, and unhealthy care of the reproductive organs, to name a few.

Some of my conversations with clients about what they learned (or didn't learn) about sexuality growing up yielded numerous themes that capture the essence of how misinformation, no information, and information acquired from peers and experience manifested for them. There were literally dozens of examples, including the following:

- I come from an older generation. My father, we never discussed anything sexual with him, the boys or the girls in my family. Sex was a dirty word; it was something you didn't talk about.

- I remember asking a lot of questions and being told "you're too young," we'll tell you when you're older, and then I went out and found out on my own. Whether it be through friends or TV, or just a lot of misinformation. But if my parents ever did have the talk with me, I had either been misinformed at that point, because I was curious before that or they explained it to me in a way that was technical and I didn't really understand it, and then I kind of learned by doing too, because I went from having my first kiss when I was 14 to having sex two months later, so there was not much of a learning curve.

- My mom and dad never really talked to me about sexuality. I lost my virginity when I was 12 years old, I was impregnated, had a kid by 14 years old. I've always been in relationships with guys and girls, that's about it.

- I learned about sexuality, let me see. On my own in the streets I guess because it wasn't talked about much at home, at all. It wasn't talked about much at school back then either. So, experiment on your own, you know that's how I learned about it.

- I was never taught, my mother never spoke about sexuality. What I learned, I learned by TV or hearing people talk about it.

Themes centered on not learning anything about sexuality from parents, learning from peers or the media, and experimentation. Noteworthy are the comments regarding shame-based messages, misinformation, and confusion. These types of messages contribute to vulnerability toward substance use and early onset of sexual behaviors. Sometimes the messages that were learned were not appropriate and were even coercive and abusive:

- Sex was never really discussed in my family. It wasn't that it was meant to be something that you didn't do; it was actually something that was very acceptable to do in my family. I started experimenting when I was 5 with the kid next door to my house who was 4 years older than me, so I knew what was going on, I learned a lot from my friends and the people I just associated myself with. And my mom, later on my mom taught me a lot of things, not how to have safe sex, but I mean she did. I remember I lost my virginity at 13, which was a miserable experience, it was humiliating. But she was the one who gave me the condoms and talked to me and told me ya know, how to, how to give blow jobs, how to do this and how to do that. My mom was a prostitute so, to me sex was something you did, sex was a way to feel loved.

- I learned about sexuality when I was at a very young age. I lost my virginity at 5 years old from my mother's boyfriend. And I figured that it was okay for a man to just do what he had to do to you and to just get it over and done with. I didn't learn about it in school because I rarely went. I was transferred from foster home to foster home, so I never really got to learn anything about sex or sexuality or how you're supposed to be with someone or anything of such nature. It was pretty bad as far as anything later on in life, that's how my addiction got even worse. Cuz I was introduced with men as far as my addiction was concerned, for me to continue my addiction I had to do sexual needs for men and women and such nature and it was just, that's how I learned, in the streets and that I just felt that it was okay to just do it with anybody just as long as I got my needs met.

In the last examples, abuse and risk for abuse were contributing factors for early onset of sex and use of substances as a coping mechanism. Inappropriate exposure to sex, dysfunctional family structures, sexual abuse, incest, and molestation were common themes in the interviews we conducted. These variables were identified by clients as directly connected to their substance-using behaviors and subsequent relapses in recovery efforts. In fact, many of the participants had never learned healthy models of sexuality and had never discussed sexuality or past sexual experiences with their counselors or any treatment providers as a rule. Other individuals shared that they had never been sober when they had sexual experiences. The last point is critical: any subsequent sexual encounter will be a relapse trigger for these clients if it is not discussed in treatment and if a relapse prevention plan does not address this factor.

EFFECTS OF LIMITED KNOWLEDGE

What we know about our bodies and how it functions, as well as our personal comfort with our bodies, can influence whether we are able to communicate with a partner, the level of risk for disease or pregnancy a person has, what to do when something is wrong, or, in some cases, having the ability to identify risk or potential problems. In some cases, the clients we interviewed said that parents (often the mothers) brought books or pamphlets home for them to read in order to learn about sexuality. For many of them, this was not enough, as they still engaged in behaviors that resulted in HIV infection, pregnancy, and vulnerability to sexual assault and molestation. Not being prepared for sexual encounters, coupled with lack of information and feelings of shame associated with engaging in sexual behaviors, is a recipe for relapse or vulnerability for substance abuse.

APPROACHES TO ASSESSING AND TEACHING ABOUT SEXUAL HEALTH

While we may not be able to definitively identify causation, the correlations are evident, and there is much we can do in terms of providing sex-positive environments for people to recover in. Suggestions for identifying what to discuss with clients in terms of reproductive and anatomical information include assessment to determine what knowledge levels exist. Determining what information is needed to fill the gaps can assist counselors in deciding what to teach rather than spending time on a topic that the group already has adequate knowledge of.

When agencies provide rote programming without the consideration client assessment, the efficacy of learning and behavior change is diminished. For example, when I worked in New York State, the state mandate for HIV education in drug and alcohol programs stated that everyone who went through treatment would receive HIV education as part of that process. So, if a client went through treatment five times, they received the same HIV overview five times. I asked myself, how does hearing the same information over and over again help individuals acquire more sophisticated skills building and information to help them stay safe unless they can be part of a more advanced group? When HIV prevention programming is offered as only a basic, one-size-fits-all course, those who have prior knowledge are left sitting in a group that is not challenging them to learn new information or to help them learn how to role-play condom use, identify personal bias or attitudes toward safer sex, or develop a personal plan for healthy behavior change.

When we consider how we are presenting information and facilitating sexuality groups through assessment, interventions can be tailored to specific group needs. With managed care, less time in treatment is a real concern for managing treatment, prioritizing needs, and providing effective services. When there is less time to work with clients, the need for the most efficacious programs becomes more critical, so, on the basis of these premises, I advocate for the use of multilevel interventions. Manualized treatment approaches should include a variety of basic, advanced, and focused lessons to provide more depth to client learning and comprehension.

THE BIGGER PICTURE

When we view sexuality broadly, there is much to consider in teaching about sexual health. Biology represents a fraction of the wheel; depending on how you slice it up, there are many areas contained on each spoke of the wheel besides that overarching theme. What good does knowing about menstruation, pregnancy, disease, and safer sex do if we have no skill or knowledge about how to apply the information to sexual situations? Does knowing how to use a condom mean we will use one? Does knowing how to use a condom help someone learn how to negotiate using it with a partner? Does knowing how a woman gets pregnant mean she will be able to choose to prevent it if she has intercourse? Does having knowledge of safer sex keep a person HIV negative? We know that knowledge alone is not a good predictor of changing health behavior. Two other key components in education include affect and skills building.

Affect has to do with how we feel about something—the attitudes, feelings, and values we have. So, if we are talking about condom use and a person has a negative attitude about using them, we may need a different approach in persuading them that they might benefit from using them. It is imperative to incorporate this type of learning into sexuality programs in order to help people uncover their personal beliefs and reconsider other ideas. I refer to this as getting a person "out of their head and into their gut." When we are in our heads, we rationalize, intellectualize, and think up all kinds of ways to avoid, deny, procrastinate, ignore, or distance ourselves from the information. "That has nothing to do with me," some-one might say. "I would know if my partner had a disease," "I'm married, I'm not at risk," "My partner is a virgin," and so on. Constructing activities that provide an "aha" moment for clients helps move them forward on a continuum of change. And thinking about change is a step toward making change happen.

BEHAVIOR CHANGE, THE TRANSTHEORETICAL MODEL OF CHANGE, AND STAGES OF CHANGE

Educating clients about sexuality is a double-edged sword. On the one hand, we want to impart information that they can use to make sound decisions with regard to sexual health and relationships. On the other hand, we may also want them to change their unhealthy ideas, beliefs, and behaviors and adopt healthier sexual habits in order to stay safe. So, this is also about behavior change, and one of the long-standing models that has been used extensively over the years is the transtheoretical model of change (TTM) also known as stages of change. This model was developed in the late 1970s and 1980s for use with smoking cessation and has since been utilized successfully with numerous other health behaviors, including substance use, weight loss, HIV prevention, and more (Prochaska, DiClemente, & Norcross, 1992).

There are several reasons I am introducing this to you: (1) it is helpful to know where a client is at in the process in order to apply the most appropriate techniques in treatment; (2) we can see when a client has moved from one stage to another, thus allowing us to change tack and move into a different type of intervention/counseling approach; (3) it allows providers to enjoy success by measuring individual movement in smaller increments rather than extremes; (4) we can better assist individuals in maintaining change; (5) we can stage individuals in other areas in order to empower them by pointing out areas in their life they are having success with; and (6) it allows us to meet a people where they are at rather than expecting them to be in a stage that we think they should be in. They are where they are, and pushing too hard when they are not ready just sets up resistance, which is not conducive to therapeutic intervention.

The five stages of change are precontemplation, contemplation, preparation, action, and maintenance (Prochaska et al., 1992; see Table 4.1). *Precontemplation* is the stage at which there is no intention to change behavior in the foreseeable future. Many individuals in this stage are unaware of a problem or may be aware of a problem but are in denial of the magnitude of the issue. *Contemplation* is the stage in which people

Table 4.1   Characteristics and Approaches for Stages of Change

Stage of Change	Characteristics	Approaches
Precontemplation	Not currently considering change. Denial that a problem exists.	• Encourage reevaluation of current behavior • Encourage self-exploration, not action • Explain and personalize the risk • Provide information • Storytelling • Discuss impact of behavior on others • Offer harm reduction options
Contemplation	Ambivalent about change: "Sitting on the fence" Not considering change within the next month	• Validate lack of readiness • Clarify: decision is theirs • Encourage evaluation of pros and cons of behavior change • Identify and promote new, positive outcome expectations • Focus on ambivalence (discuss pros and cons of change and perceived barriers to change, offer substitutes/harm reduction) • Explore behaviors in relation to self-image
Preparation/ready for action	Some experience with change and are trying to change: "Testing the waters" Planning to act within one month	• Identify and assist in problem solving regarding obstacles • Develop a plan (build self-confidence, practice skills, negotiate the first step) • Help patient identify social support • Verify that patient has underlying skills for behavior change • Encourage small initial steps
Action	Practicing new behavior for three to six months	• Focus on restructuring cues and social support, identify support

(*continued*)

Table 4.1 (continued)

Stage of Change	Characteristics	Approaches
		• Bolster self-efficacy for dealing with obstacles, find substitutes • Combat feelings of loss and reiterate long-term benefits • Identify rewards • Avoid cues
Maintenance	Continued commitment to sustaining new behavior for more than six months	• Plan for follow-up support • Reinforce internal rewards • Discuss coping with relapse • Become a role model
Relapse	Resumption of old behaviors	• Evaluate trigger for relapse • Reassess motivation and barriers • Plan stronger coping strategies

Source: Adapted from Center for Health and Behavioral Training, Rochester, New York.

are aware that a problem exists and are seriously thinking about overcoming it but have not yet made a commitment to take action. One way to tell that a person is contemplative are statements that start with "Yea, but . . ." The "but" is indicative of ambivalence, and this ambivalence is what needs to be addressed. *Preparation*, or *ready for action*, is a stage that combines intention and behavioral criteria. Individuals in this stage are intending to take action in the next month. Interventions for the person who is in this stage include helping him or her make a plan. *Action* is the stage in which individuals modify their behavior, experiences, or environment in order to overcome their problems. Action involves the most overt behavioral changes and requires considerable commitment of time and energy. In a harm reduction continuum, the change may not be abstinence or extinction of a risk behavior but may be a modification of the behavior, albeit a step in a safer direction. *Maintenance* is the stage in which people work to prevent relapse and consolidate the gains attained during action. For addictive behaviors, this stage extends from six months or more past the initial action (Prochaska et al., 1992).

Another stage was added to this model, called *relapse*. Relapse is when a person has a lapse in the changed behavior that may last a day or a week, or the person may return to the past lifestyle. A person who has relapsed may go right back into action, may start to make a plan, or may cycle back to the beginning. What is difficult for people to grasp, particularly with substance use, is that relapse is normal and a part of the process. Seven seems to be the magic number. As with most behavior change (e.g., going on a diet, working out, or eating healthy), individuals will relapse on average seven times before they get it right: some more, some less. The interesting thing about substance users is that many people look down on them and judge them more harshly than if they were trying to reduce their cholesterol and went to McDonald's and binged on some greasy food. Substance use is a behavior, like any other behavior, and the sooner we can put that into perspective, the better we will serve our clients with less judgment.

The stages of change address a facet of behavior change ignored by many other theories, namely, that change is a process that occurs over time. The stages are also not linear, and while they may occur in a linear fashion, a nonlinear progression is more common. A person may move through them, skipping stages, or recycle back and forth between different ones several times. It is helpful to know this because if the client is moving back and forth, we can be assured that this is normal and adjust our intervention techniques accordingly. Using this model helped me enormously in my HIV work. I had clients who were all over the place in terms of their adherence to medications, substance use, and HIV risk with partners and more. They cannot do it all overnight, and if they recycle through the stages, that does not mean they are a failure. If we can be there to help them move forward and not act punitively, we will go far in empowering them to create and maintain positive change in their lives. Change often comes at its own pace—often quickly and in bursts rather than a consistent rate. It is not unusual for someone to spend years in precontemplation and then progress to action in a matter of weeks or months.

The prior examples given clients in "denial" denotes the stage of precontemplation, and the "aha" moment is the shift from precontemplation to contemplation. Now that person is considering the information; something that was presented helped that client consider change. It may have been a story that brought it home to them or an activity that got them to connect with the information. Active teaching allows people to interact with what you are presenting and grapple with what it means or how it might impact them. This typically does not happen in a pure lecture format.

Three other components of TTM characterize its internal workings: decisional balance, self-efficacy, and processes of change (Prochaska et al., 1992). Decision making was conceptualized as a decisional "balance sheet" of comparative potential gains and losses. Two components of decisional balance, the pros and the cons, have become critical constructs in TTM. As individuals progress through the stages of change, decisional balance shifts in critical ways. When an individual is in the pre-contemplation stage, the pros in favor of behavioral change are out-weighed by the relative cons for change and in favor of maintaining the existing behavior. In the precontemplation stage, the pros and cons tend to carry equal weight, leaving the individual ambivalent toward change. If the decisional balance is tipped, however, such that the pros in favor of changing outweigh the cons for maintaining the unhealthy behavior, many individuals move to the preparation or even the action stage. As individuals enter the maintenance stage, the pros in favor of maintaining the behavioral change should outweigh the cons of maintaining the change in order to decrease the risk of relapse.

Stages of change integrate elements of Albert Bandura's (1977, 1982) self-efficacy theory. This construct reflects the degree of confidence the individual has in maintaining his or her desired behavioral change in sit-uations that often trigger relapse. It is also measured by the degree to which the individual feels tempted to return to his or her problem behavior in these high-risk situations. If a client does not feel confident in his or her ability to change, this can impede the process. In the precontemplation and contemplation stages, an individual's temptation to engage in the problem behavior is far greater than his or her self-efficacy to abstain. As the individual moves from preparation to action, the disparity between feelings of self-efficacy and temptation closes, and behavioral change is attained. Relapse often occurs in situations where feelings of temptation trump an individual's sense of self-efficacy to maintain the desired behav-ioral change.

Processes of Change

While the stages of change are useful in explaining when changes in cognition, emotion, and behavior take place, the processes of change help to explain how these changes occur. These 10 processes need to be imple-mented to successfully progress through the stages of change and attain the desired behavioral change. The processes can be divided into two groups: cognitive and affective experiential processes and behavioral pro-cesses (see Table 4.2).

Let's say that one day you wake up, and in the news the surgeon general has announced that watching television causes brain cancer. How many of you would turn off your television and get rid of it on hearing this news? In a room of 30 people, a handful of people might move right into action. Many people will remain in a state of denial or contemplation, needing

Table 4.2   Stages of Change Processes

Experiential	• *Consciousness raising*—Knowledge and awareness about the individual and their problem behavior is increased. • *Dramatic relief*—Emotions about the individual's problem behavior and available treatments or solutions are aroused. • *Environmental reevaluation*—The impact that the individual's problem behavior has on his or her environment is reassessed. • *Self-reevaluation*—Cognitions and emotions regarding the individual, especially with respect to his or her problem behavior, are reassessed. • *Self-liberation*—Choosing a course of action to change the problem behavior and committing to that choice.
Behavioral	• *Reinforcement management*—Positive behavioral changes are rewarded. • *Helping relationships*—Trusting and open discussion about the problem behavior is received by a supporting individual(s). • *Counterconditioning*—Positive alternative behaviors are substituted for the individual's problem behavior. • *Stimulus control*—Stimuli that may trigger lapse back to the problem behavior are prepared to be coped with, removed, or avoided. • *Social liberation*—Attempts are made to decrease the prevalence of the individual's former problem behavior in society.

more evidence before they decide to move to another stage. Now, let's say that a year has passed, and there are preliminary results from studies that document the claim; we now have pictures of diseased brains from control studies comparing them to brains of people who have quit watching television, and the images show clear improvement in brain matter. How many more of you would move to another stage? In that same group of people, a few might shift to contemplative or even action, while those who already quit would move into maintenance. What if a close family member were stricken with the television-based brain cancer? Would this prompt any more of you to consider change?

This is basically how the process works. In each stage, we can ask questions, provide information, and develop methods to help a person move from one stage to another. For some people, it takes time and more information. For others, it may take a personal event to affect their decision to change. Of course, this is a simplistic example, but it is intended to give you an idea of how it works. Everyone has their own bottom line or situation that shifts the balance to change.

Sex and Behavior Change

What does all this have to do with sex? When we are counseling or running groups and working with sexuality issues, being able to "stage" individuals (or even groups of people) helps us move them forward and apply appropriate interventions and techniques. There are many issues around sexual anatomy and physiology as well as the other areas that will come up over the course of providing sexuality information and running sexual health groups. Incorporating TTM as a strategy will aid us in providing effective interventions and in matching the intervention appropriately to the group's needs.

CONNECTIONS TO SUBSTANCE USE

In terms of sexual anatomy and functioning related to substance use, there are a number of issues that may influence a person's decision to use. Some of these include clients who are experiencing reproductive disorders and who therefore cannot easily become parents. Other physiological issues include impotency for men, sexual dysfunction, infertility (both for men and women), or other disorders related to the care and function of the reproductive system. For some people, when they experience the loss of the ability to be sexual with a partner, have erections, have an orgasm, have children, or be disease free, they experience not only loss of potential partners and intimacy but also loss of feeling like a "man" or a "woman" based on traditional gender role socialization. These feelings can be accompanied by a sense of shame and loss of self-worth, and, in order to cope or numb the feelings, alcohol or substance use may end up as a surrogate partner.

Studies on women with reproductive dysfunction found that they deal with such problems in a variety of ways, including the use of alcohol and other drugs to dull the emotional pain and loss (Gomberg, 1994). A significant relationship has been demonstrated between miscarriages and hysterectomies on the one hand and heavy drinking among alcoholic women in treatment on the other (Gomberg, 1994). Several women we interviewed expressed direct connections to their infertility and miscarriages to substance-using behaviors:

Lisa: I put feelings and attitudes and the physiology and anatomy of reproductive organs because I had a miscarriage with like one of my boyfriends and I wasn't using at the time and we was doing everything right. And so after that, we tried to get pregnant for a whole year after that and I was like okay, maybe I can't have kids. And then things didn't work out with him, I got another boyfriend, and we was together for two years and we tried getting pregnant and I had another miscarriage, and so after that I just grew really depressed, I was like okay I'm never gonna have kids, I really went into a depression after my miscarriages, and started using a lot more, it really affected me as a woman because I felt like I couldn't have kids.

Mandy: Before I ever started drinking or using or anything, I was married and we had tried to have kids and I couldn't get pregnant and it just seemed to be kind of or part of why our marriage didn't last. Towards the end of our marriage I started drinking a little and then after I left him, I was drinking enormous amounts. And I don't know, I just, every time I was in a relationship, I was hoping okay maybe I'll get pregnant this time. Every pregnancy scare that didn't turn out, it just turned back into either drinking and then after I started using heroin, it wasn't even, I didn't even care about that anymore. I was done with that, I just, I didn't even want to be touched. I had boyfriends that, long-term boyfriends that I wouldn't even let sleep in the same bed with me.

Being able to help clients identify these connections is critical for healing to take place. Those clients who identify reproductive issues as connected to their substance misuse and relapse, whether it is infertility, abortion, miscarriage, impotency, or sexual dysfunction, need to have avenues for exploring the feelings and behaviors associated with them. And this leads us right back to having sexual health counselors as part of the team. Some agencies utilize outside entities, such as Planned Parenthood or the local health department, to provide such information. But outsourcing for all of our program's sexuality-related programming does nothing to increase the comfort and knowledge base of existing staff and counselors. It makes sense to minimally have a person or two on board who can facilitate a variety of sexuality groups and to train other staff to conduct groups. Once a team of trained sexual health counselors exists in a program, the turnover of staff will not affect continuity of services. The more the merrier when it comes to talking about sex.

SEXUAL DYSFUNCTIONS AND THEIR TREATMENT

In addition to reproductive functioning, anatomy and physiology is another area of the blue-light special that often goes unaddressed in sexual health programming; this relates to sexual dysfunction. For those who are vulnerable to using or who use substances, there are many links to this facet of sexual health. Often, individuals may use certain chemicals in the hope of enhancing sexual pleasure or to "treat" their own depression resulting from sexual dysfunction.

Human Sexual Response

In order to understand how these disorders are linked, some background on sexual functioning is pertinent. William Masters and Virginia Johnson were major contributors to understanding the process of human sexual response through thousands of hours of extensive laboratory research during the 1950s and 1960s. The resulting model of physiological response described four stages: (1) excitement, (2) plateau, (3) orgasm, and (4) resolution. Their model documents genital and extragenital changes that typically occur in each of these changes (see Figure 4.1).

In the decade following Masters and Johnson's (1966) famous publication *Human Sexual Response*, it became clear that something was missing from the model, as many sexually troubled individuals had complaints about lack of interest or desire as well as aversions to sexual activities. This preliminary phase was subsequently labeled "sexual desire." Sexual desire involves "a person's readiness for, and interest in, sexual activity" (Wincze & Carey, 2001, p. 4). The physiological and subjective arousal for sexual activity and subsequent orgasm were much less likely to occur without sexual desire.

Types of Sexual Dysfunction

Today, most sexologists agree that healthy sexual functioning involves three primary stages: desire, arousal, and orgasm. Sexual dysfunctions can be categorized under four major areas: (1) sexual desire disorders, (2) sexual arousal disorders, (3) orgasmic disorders, and (4) sexual pain disorders; they consist of impairment or disturbance in one of the primary stages. There are also nine major diagnostic categories in the *Diagnostic and Statistical Manual of Mental Disorders* (4th ed., text revision), Although the manual was developed for mental health care professionals, these categories and criteria address the most commonly seen sexual difficulties (see Table 4.3).

Figure 4.1   Courtesy of WebMD.

Human Sexual Response Cycle

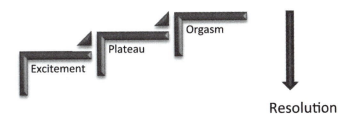

The sexual response cycle has four phases: excitement, plateau, orgasm, and resolution. Both men and women experience these phases, although the timing usually is different. For example, it is unlikely that both partners will reach orgasm at
the same time. In addition, the intensity of the response and the time spent in each
phase varies from person to person. Understanding these differences may help
partners better understand one another's bodies and responses, and enhance the
sexual experience.

Phase 1: Excitement. General characteristics of the excitement phase, which can
last from a few minutes to several hours, include the following:

Muscle tension increases, heart rate quickens and breathing is accelerated, skin
may become flushed (blotches of redness appear on the chest and back), nipples
become hardened or erect, blood flow to the genitals increases, resulting in swell-
ing of the woman's clitoris and labia minora (inner lips), and erection of the
man's penis, vaginal lubrication begins, the woman's breasts become fuller and
the vaginal walls begin to swell, the man's testicles swell, his scrotum tightens,
and he begins secreting a lubricating liquid.

Phase 2: Plateau. General characteristics of the plateau phase, which extends to
the brink of orgasm, include the following:

The changes begun in phase 1 are intensified, the vagina continues to swell from
increased blood flow, and the vaginal walls turn a dark purple, the woman's clitoris
becomes highly sensitive (may even be painful to touch) and retracts under the
clitoral hood to avoid direct stimulation from the penis, the man's testicles are
withdrawn up into the scrotum, breathing, heart rate, and blood pressure continue
to increase, muscle spasms may begin in the feet, face, and hands, muscle tension
increases.

Phase 3: Orgasm. The orgasm is the climax of the sexual response cycle. It is the shortest of the phases and generally lasts only a few seconds. General characteristics of this phase include the following:

Involuntary muscle contractions begin, blood pressure, heart rate, and breathing are at their highest rates, with a rapid intake of oxygen, muscles in the feet spasm, there is a sudden, forceful release of sexual tension. In women, the muscles of the vagina contract and the uterus also undergoes rhythmic contractions. In men, rhythmic contractions of the muscles at the base of the penis result in the ejaculation of semen. A rash, or "sex flush" may appear over the entire body.

Phase 4: Resolution. During resolution, the body slowly returns to its normal level of functioning, and swelled and erect body parts return to their previous size and color. This phase is marked by a general sense of well-being, enhanced intimacy and, often, fatigue. Some women are capable of a rapid return to the orgasm phase with further sexual stimulation and may experience multiple orgasms. Men need recovery time after orgasm, called a refractory period, during which they cannot reach orgasm again. The duration of the refractory period varies among men and usually lengthens with advancing age.

From: http://www.webmd.com/sex-relationships/guide/sexual-health-your -guide-to-sexual-response-cycle

---

When we examine the causes of sexual dysfunctions, classifications can be viewed as medical or biological, hormonal (due to changes across the life span), or psychological. Major depression and other anxiety disorders are commonly associated with problems of sexual functioning. Other contributing psychological causes include negative body image and fear of rejection or negative reactions (Wincze & Carey, 2001). Sexual abuse or other health conditions can increase vulnerability to problems with sexual functioning, and everyday stress can trigger problems as well. Sexual dysfunctions are common, and with the introduction of Viagra as a treatment for erectile dysfunction came the permission to seek assistance for the treatment and legitimization of sexual dysfunctions as a medical entity.

Of course, the complex associations between assessment, identification, and treatment are beyond the scope of this text and perhaps the substance abuse realm. However, we need to have knowledge of how this area is intimately linked to the lives of our clients and not ignore the magnitude of impact that sexual dysfunction can have on an individual's existence. Simply giving a person medication to treat any disorder does not always "fix" the problem. Delving into the underlying connections to experiences,

Table 4.3   Categories of Sexual Dysfunction among Men and Women

Phase of Response Cycle Affected	Men	Women
Desire	Hypoactive sexual desire disorder	Hypoactive sexual desire disorder
	Sexual aversion disorder	Sexual aversion disorder
Arousal	Male erectile disorder	Female sexual arousal disorder
Orgasm	Male orgasmic disorder	Female orgasmic disorder
	Premature ejaculation	
Pain	Dyspareunia	Dyspareunia
		Vaginismus

Source: Adapted from Wincze and Carey (2001).

physical health, relational dynamics, and so on will go a long way in helping us to properly refer folks to appropriate treatment and resources.

TREATMENT APPROACHES

Presentations about sexuality, menstruation, birth control, pregnancy, and childbirth to empower women with knowledge of the choices available to them are advocated (Volpe & Hamilton, 1982–1983). Fostering sexual autonomy in female clients by helping them identify and express their sexual desires, preferences, and limits as a means of addressing and healing the effects of abuse is encouraged (Mumme, 1991). We know that women in treatment respond well to gender-specific interventions that include discussions of HIV, sexuality, communication, and sexual health concerns (Bartholomew, Rowan-Szal, Chatham, & Simpson, 1994; Camp & Finkelstein, 1997). Self-esteem, intimacy, and sexuality were identified as central issues for men in recovery, but men often have difficulty acknowledging their needs, fears, and concerns in these areas because of male gender role socialization (Norwinski, 1993). Men's and women's concerns regarding sexual dysfunctions also need to be addressed in order for them to achieve acceptable levels of sexual satisfaction.

Developing and implementing sexual health programming in treatment will assist clients in managing issues related to these identified areas. Whether we use existing programming or train staff and counselors to develop curricula, offering programs to clients as a regular part of treatment is clearly indicated to help prevent subsequent relapse, keep them in treatment, and provide them with skills and information to stay safe, take care of their bodies, and live a more sexually healthy life. Programs that include and address issues associated with the genitals and reproductive systems, birth control, abortion issues, infertility, impotency, and sexual dysfunction will aid clients in understanding how these areas impact their attitudes toward substance use and their ability to make informed decisions, minimize risk outcomes, and find treatment and therapy to help them move past pain and to heal without having to rely on substances.

COMMUNITY PARTNERSHIPS

This is no small undertaking, so being knowledgeable about community resources is one way you can help. Find out who the qualified sex therapists are in your area who specialize in areas of infertility or sexual dysfunctions. Know which medical providers are knowledgeable in assessing for sexual dysfunction. Become educated in matters of birth control and comfortable in discussing abortion and emergency contraception. Read up on sexual dysfunctions and their treatments. Having a broad foundation of knowledge gives you the ability to provide direction and to help clients include sexual health issues in their treatment plans.

GENDER DIFFERENCES

We also want to make sure that we have men-only and women-only group options available to conduct sexual health programming. This is optimal, not required. Some programs have conducted mixed-gender groups for sexual health with good results (Braun-Harvey, 2009). Concerns associated with mixed-gender groups include (1) the revictimization of women by men (or vice versa), which can trigger past trauma; (2) sexual tension in the group, which can create unnecessary distractions; (3) women and men having different experiences with their sexuality and addiction, so programming for women may not be on target for what men are dealing with; (4) the facilitator not being sensitive in dealing with gender differences and inadvertently leaving clients vulnerable from the dynamics of a particular group or topic; and (5) fear of client expression due to socialized gender roles, as when a man discloses sexual abuse in a group of women.

In the event that your program is not large enough for gender-specific groups, you can provide one-on-one sessions as needed or run small specialty groups. We know that mixed-gender treatment programs are comprised predominantly of men, so it would be easier to form some male-only sexual health groups. The key is to make sure that topics represent the needs of the men in the group. There may be times when combining groups could work to your benefit; for example, a male relationship group practicing skills building might be able to team up with some female partners for practice, or a women's group might benefit from eliciting a male perspective on a chosen topic. As long as care is taken to protect the individuals in the groups, creativity in developing programming will keep it fresh and interesting.

SAMPLE BIRTH CONTROL LESSON

This particular topic can be included as part of a sexual health curriculum. If we are including birth control information as part of a sexual health group, it might follow a lesson on safer sex, relationships, or even as part of an adolescent group.

Goal: Through the use of a matching activity and small-group discussion, participants will learn about pregnancy prevention methods and how to best apply these methods to their sexual relationships.

Rationale: Issues related to pregnancy prevention can be indirectly related to substance abuse. Some individuals have experienced emotional pain through the loss of their children due to neglect or abuse in the home and may benefit from preventing further pregnancies until they feel able to handle the responsibility of having another child. Others may have experienced emotional pain due to multiple pregnancies and abortion, unwanted pregnancies, or forced pregnancies by a partner and may need information to help them prevent further traumatic experiences. Being able to understand family planning options can help participants gain control over their lives if they have experienced a loss of control through misunderstanding reproductive health.

Time: 90 minutes

Objectives: Participants will do the following:

- Identify multiple methods of birth control
- Distinguish between hormonal, barrier, and natural family planning methods
- Identify the efficacy of several methods
- Assess which methods might be best
- Discuss possible options for negotiating birth control in a relationship

Materials:

- List of birth control methods (Appendix C) cut out and taped on index cards (facilitator should have several sets; each set should be on a separate color index card to distinguish between sets, so one on blue cards, another on red, and so on)
- Fact sheet (sample): http://www.cdc.gov/reproductivehealth/ UnintendedPregnancy/Contraception.htm
- Index cards labeled "hormonal," "barrier," "natural," and "permanent" (these cards should be taped on a wall prior to the start of the group, leaving a couple of feet of space between cards)
- Case studies: http://www.kingcounty.gov/healthservices/health/ personal/famplan/educators/~/media/health/publichealth/documents/ famplan/G910_L22.ashx
- Masking tape
- Newsprint, markers
- Pretest/posttest

Procedure:
Birth Control Methods (45 minutes)

1. Introduce the topic, distribute the pretest, and ask that they complete the survey. Facilitator can also read the questions to the group in the event any participants have trouble reading. Collect the pretests.

2. Ask participants what facts they know about birth control. Elicit some responses from the group and record responses on a whiteboard or newsprint. Ask the group why they think this topic could be important in their recovery (record responses). Based on recorded responses, validate their comments and tell them which areas you will be addressing in the program today, providing some rationale for doing so.

3. Break the large group into smaller groups of about three to five participants each. Optimally, no more than three groups should exist; two groups are also acceptable. Pass out the index cards with the birth control methods/pictures. Each group should have a full set of all the methods. Instruct each group to decide among themselves which of the methods they have are either barrier, natural, or a hormonal method. Instruct them to tape their cards on the wall

under the matching category when their group has processed the methods.

4. Once the groups have taped their cards to the wall according to category, ask them to view the other sets of cards and give them a few minutes to decide if they wish to move any of their methods to a different category. After this is completed, one person from each group should remain at the wall.

5. Next, the facilitator should ask one of the groups to list which methods they posted under hormonal methods. After that participant has read off their list, the facilitator should correct any mismatched methods, and each group member should readjust his or her cards. Repeat this step with a participant from another group reading off their list until all categories are covered and corrected. Using the fact sheet, the facilitator should discuss basic information related to each method, their effectiveness and associated costs, and any related medical procedures during this process.

Process questions include the following:

- Were there any methods that you had difficulty in placing? Which ones and why?
- Were there any methods you were not familiar with? Which ones?
- Which methods would you feel most comfortable using and why?
- Would your choice change if you were in a relationship with another person versus if you were not in a relationship? Why or why not?
- How might the relationship factor impact your ability to effectively manage family planning?

Case Study (45 minutes)
Using the last process question regarding the relationship factor, introduce the next activity. Having information can help us only if we are able to apply it to real-life situations. The following case studies will provide us with tools that will enable us to apply the information to several real-life situations as well as our own.

1. Once each method is processed, give each participant a handout that describes each method, costs, and efficacy. Provide each group with a case study and the "Real Person's Decisions" worksheet. Have the groups work together to determine how effectiveness, cost, protection

against sexually transmitted infections, medical conditions, and beliefs impact the decision-making process for the case involved.

2. Allow about 20 minutes for each group to assess and evaluate their case, then process each case in the large group. The facilitator should encourage discussion and relate the factors assessment to group members' personal decision-making regarding family planning.

3. Administer the posttest after completing process

4. A homework assignment might include a journal activity that asks participants to discuss how they felt about the session and the learning or an assignment that asks them to develop their personal scenario and then apply the factors and decision-making process to themselves. The homework could be used for individual treatment planning if there are concerns directly related to substance use or relapse concerns.

Every time I teach a group of students or clients or professionals about a sexuality topic, that group brings their own ideas, bias, understanding, and experiences to the table. With this comes my challenge. The more methods and activities I have at my disposal, the better able I am to effectively provide them with what they need. I often overplan; that is, I bring more activities than I need in case I have to change direction based on their needs. Some of these ideas reside in my head and do not take many extra materials, but thinking ahead helps us to think on our feet once we have gained some experience teaching and facilitating. As far as having the extras lurking in our heads, that comes with time and practice. In the meantime, utilize the resources for access to plenty of awesome lesson plans and to enhance your learning.

REPRODUCTIVE RESOURCES

Books

Boston Women's Health Collective. (2010). *Our bodies, ourselves.* Boston: Boston Women's Health Collective.

Herbenick, D., & Schick, V. (2011). *Read my lips: A complete guide to the vagina and vulva.* New York: Rowman & Littlefield.

McCarthy, B. W., & Metz, M. E. (2008). *Men's sexual health: Fitness for satisfying sex.* New York: Routledge.

Online Resources

Anatomy of Sex. http://topdocumentaryfilms.com/anatomy-sex. This free online documentary travels inside the body to see what happens when attraction, orgasm, and reproduction occur in the human body.

The Clitoris.com. http://www.the-clitoris.com. This website is dedicated to female sexual pleasure and health. It provides resources related to anatomy, sexual functioning, and orgasm.

Our Bodies Ourselves. http://www.ourbodiesourselves.org. This website provides information about sexual anatomy and reproduction as well as blogs about sexuality and sexually transmitted infections.

Planned Parenthood. http://www.plannedparenthood.org/health-topics/sex-101/reproductive-sexual-anatomy-22959.htm.

3dvulva. http://www.3dvulva.com. This website provides diagrams of the vulva, clitoris, labia, and other female sex organs.

FIVE

Taking Care of Business and Safer Sex

Remember when safe sex meant not getting caught?

—Anonymous

Sexual health in the realm of safer sex encompasses a number of issues, including self-care of the genitals (pap smears for women and testicular self-exams for men), knowledge of and use of barriers to prevent disease, knowing one's body and how to respond appropriately when issues arise, and being able to attend to physical changes and obtain regular testing for sexually transmitted infections (STIs) and HIV when appropriate. Along with the need for being able to know one's body as discussed in the previous chapter, people need to be able to become comfortable with their bodies in order to care for them. If I am uncomfortable with my body, I am not likely to check my breasts regularly for lumps or to discuss or notice changes in my partner's body as well. And if I am ashamed or embarrassed about my body, I may subsequently put myself at risk for disease as a result.

We can see evidence of people's discomfort in the language they use when referring to their genitals or the genitals of others. We hear euphemisms such as "down there," "going downtown," "snatch," "cootchie," "johnson," and more to describe genitalia rather than the actual anatomical names of body parts. Why are the words "vagina," "penis," "labia," "clitoris," and "testicles" so embarrassing to say? As a counselor or health care worker, examining our discomfort is critical in order to provide accurate and understandable information and care to clients.

STIs

In this chapter, a variety of STIs (formerly known as sexually transmitted diseases) are discussed, as are strategies for prevention and sexual discussion. The shift in terminology to "STI" resulted from the mind-set that many of these infections are not diseases and that the term "infection" more accurately and inclusively describes their etiology (causes). "STI" is the terminology that is used in this chapter.

The United States has the highest rate of STIs of any industrialized nation. Sexually active youth in the United States account for about half of all the new cases of annual infections. More than half of all Americans will get an STI at some point in their lifetime (American Social Health Association, 2005).

STIs have been in existence for centuries. Some of these infections are curable (bacterial); others are not (viral). With the growing rates of STIs and the emergence of new types of viral infections over the last few decades, the implications for treatment and prevention of STIs have become more complex and frustrating for educators and providers alike.

Most individuals will present with sexual risk and infection over the course of their lives. The information presented here is intended to assist readers in making informed decisions about sexual choices they are likely to encounter and in talking to sexual partners about STIs, testing, and prevention. This important process of knowledge and intervention is crucial for initiating, developing, and maintaining healthy relationships and lifestyles.

PREVALENCE OF STIs

The Centers for Disease Control (CDC, 2004) estimates that 19 million new infections occur each year, almost half of them among young people ages 15 to 24 (2004). The number of documented AIDS cases in the United States is over 900,000 with approximately 40,000 new HIV infections each year (CDC, 2004). Although AIDS diagnosis and deaths are lower than in previous times, the decrease has to do more with treatment intervention than with rates of infection. STIs and HIV disproportionately impact the health of African Americans and Latinos as compared with whites. Here is a brief summary of some STI statistics in the United States:

- In 2009, a total of 1,244,180 cases of sexually transmitted chlamydia infection were reported to the CDC. This is the largest number of cases ever reported to the CDC for any condition (CDC, 2009).

- Gonorrhea is the second most commonly reported infectious disease in the United States, with 301,174 cases reported in 2009 (CDC, 2009a).

- In 2009, a total of 13,997 cases of primary and secondary syphilis were reported to the CDC. This case count is the highest number of cases reported since 1995. Since 2005, the rate of primary and secondary syphilis has increased 59 percent (CDC, 2009b).

- In total, the CDC estimates that there are approximately 19 million new sexually transmitted diseases infections each year (CDC, 2009c).

Despite of the high incidence of STIs, knowledge levels are low in adolescents, adults, and their health care providers. Continuing to ignore the existence and risk of STIs will not make the problem disappear. By educating students and other health care professionals and ourselves, we can help find ways to intervene, prevent, and treat STIs.

Many factors contribute to the epidemic of STIs in the United States. Having multiple partners and sexual contact with no barriers is a major reason for the high incidence of STIs in adolescence and early adulthood (Feroli & Burstein, 2003). Lack of adequate public health measures and limited access to treatment also contribute to this major health problem. It is common for physicians and nurse practitioners to be reluctant to ask questions about their patients' sexual behaviors and thereby to lose opportunities for STI-related counseling, diagnosis, and treatment. A nationally representative survey of 3,390 U.S. adults ages 18 to 64 found that only 28 percent reported being asked about STIs during routine medical checkups (Tao, Irvine, & Kassler, 2000). Another national survey that examined sex, alcohol, and STIs found that problematic drinking among men and women can increase the risk for STI (Erikson & Trocki, 1994).

The majority of persons with STIs are asymptomatic (have no symptoms) and unaware of their infections. This contributes to the spread of STIs. Commonly, women and men will not experience any symptoms despite having an infection. In this instance, a person may unknowingly infect another person with a STI. Often, infected individuals are embarrassed to seek treatment or talk to their partner about being infected, exacerbating the situation. In the prevention section of this chapter, we will learn tips for talking to a partner about STIs as well as tips for safer sex practices.

STIs can be broken down into two main categories: bacterial and viral. Bacterial STIs are curable; they more commonly include chlamydia, gonorrhea, syphilis (first and second stage), trichomoniasis, and nongonoccocal urethritis. Viral STIs are incurable, although antiviral drugs are being developed at this time to treat symptoms of viral infections. Viral STIs include HIV, herpes, hepatitis, and human papillomavirus, or genital warts. Causes, symptoms and complications, diagnosis, and treatments regarding the infections are provided in more detail on the CDC's website. If you need more information, it is recommended that you contact your local health department or call the CDC. This information can be located in the listing of resources at the end of this chapter. These services can answer questions, provide free literature, or refer you to a local clinic for testing and treatment. Tables 5.1 and 5.2 give brief overviews of symptoms and treatment for the most common STIs (a separate chart is provided for HIV disease progression).

HIV

HIV is not included in the previous tables for several reasons. First, although HIV can be sexually transmitted, it can also be contracted in other ways (mother to fetus or infant or exposure to infected blood, such as through fighting, accidents, and sharing needles). Next, the incubation period is misleading in the tables. You are either infected or not after having risk for exposure. The window period refers to the length of time after infection before an accurate HIV test can be confirmed. After infection, it can take between one and three months for a person's body to summon an immune response. An HIV test confirms that *antibodies* for HIV are present; it does not test for the actual virus. And the way in which HIV impacts the immune system actually slows down the immune response through the white blood cells it infects (T4 or CD4 cells and macrophages, key players in mounting the immune response). Incubation and infection is not the same thing; incubation has to do with the time an infection occurs and when signs and symptoms appear, which in the case of HIV can take an average of 10 years.

Even though HIV infection takes so long to manifest symptoms, great damage is being wreaked on the immune system. Once HIV enters the body, it infects CD4 cells, and billions of viruses can be produced daily; once the immune system responds, billions of viruses can effectively be destroyed through effective antibody production. This "silent" war can progress more rapidly if negative cofactors to disease progression are present, such as drug and alcohol use, poor nutrition, other infections, smoking, stress, and so on. Thus, when we consider disease progression, length of time to symptoms and diseases, and substance abuse, the person who is infected but is not aware of the infection poses a great risk to others. There are estimated to be at least four times as many people

Table 5.1 Common Viral STIs: Symptoms and Treatment

Infection/Cause	Symptoms	Transmission	Incubation Period	Treatments	Complications
Human papilloma virus (HPV) Estimated 40 to 60 percent warts are flat type, showing no symptoms.	W&M: Florid (visible) warts range from small, slightly raised bumps to larger, rough-textured bumps. Flat (nonvisible) warts create changes in cell structure that can be seen only with certain clinical tests. May itch. Occur on penis, labia, vagina, cervix, and anus.	Vaginal and anal intercourse. Actively infected mother to trachea of newborn.	Three weeks to 8 months average but can be up to 18 to 20 months.	No known cure for virus; warts may recur; specific wart infections can be treated by various methods, depending on site and type of wart, including cryosurgery and topical treatments. If warts are anal, get HIV test.	Certain strains may increase risk of cervical cancer in women; not known if cancer risk is increased for men.
Herpes simplex virus (HSV I and HSV II) Estimated that two-thirds of herpes cases may be transmitted unknowingly during incubation because of	W&M: Before outbreak: itching, tingling, sensitivity in area, flu-like symptoms. Outbreak: Blister-type sore breaks open to	Vaginal and anal intercourse. Oral-oral contact; oral-genital-anal contact. Actively infected mother to newborn.	5 to 21 days.	No known cure; oral acyclovir used to suppress frequent outbreaks. If sores are anal or if acyclovir does not	Serious only for pregnant women; if first outbreak occurs while pregnant, can cause premature delivery; recurrence during

(continued)

Table 5.1 (continued)

Infection/Cause	Symptoms	Transmission	Incubation Period	Treatments	Complications
misdiagnosis, atypical symptoms, or shedding of virus when some sores are not present or visible.	leave raw, painful area; scabs over. Occurs on mouth, penis, labia, vagina, cervix, and anus.			control recurrences, get HIV test.	delivery; can infect newborn.
Viral hepatitis (HAV, HBV, HCV, *HDV, HEV) Inflammation of the liver caused by a virus. Can be short term or long term. Hepatitis B, C, and D viruses can cause chronic (long-term) hepatitis.	W&M: Symptoms include jaundice, fatigue, stomach pain, and nausea. Some forms of hepatitis go away on their own, while others require medical treatment.	HAV and HEV: Spread through fecal-oral transmission, sex, and household contact. HBV: Spread through contact with infected blood or bodily fluids. HCV: Transmitted through infected blood and sharing infected needles and from mother to infant during childbirth. Rarely through sexual intercourse.	HAV and HEV: 15 to 50 days; average 28 days. HBV: 45 to 160 days; average 120 days. HCV: 14 to 180 days; average 45 days.	Bed rest, interferon, pegylated interferon, other antiviral medications, liver transplant. No known cure; some forms of viral hepatitis will clear the body over time, while other forms will progress to chronic stages.	Most HAV infections clear within six months; HBV, HCV, HDV, or HEV can progress to chronic illness, resulting in liver failure, liver cancer, and death.

*HDV cannot be contracted unless the person is already infected with HBV.

Note: W = women; M = men; W&M = women and men.

Source: Adapted from: http://www.immunize.org/catg.d/p4075abc.pdf and http://www.birth-control-comparison.info/bc_pdf/sti_chart.pdf.

Table 5.2 Common Bacterial STIs: Symptoms and Treatment

Infection/Cause	Symptoms	Transmission	Incubation Period	Treatments	Complications
Chlamydia (*Chlamydia trachomatis bacteria*)	W: Vaginal discharge, irregular bleeding, irritation in urethra, PID symptoms; two-thirds have no symptoms. M: Penile discharge, itching, burning; one-third have no symptoms.	Vaginal and anal intercourse.	7 to 21 days.	Oral antibiotics; treat partners, use condom.	PID for women; sterility. Epididymitis/prostatis/arthritis for men.
Gonorrhea (*Neisseria gonorrhea bacteria*)	W: Vaginal discharge, irregular bleeding, PID symptoms; 25 to 50 percent have no symptoms. M: Penile, anal discharge, burning, itching; 5 to 10 percent have no symptoms.	Vaginal and anal intercourse; Oral-genital (throat infections for receiver of penis).	2 to 7 days.	Oral antibiotics; treat partners, use condom.	PID for women; sterility. Epididymitis/prostatis/arthritis for men.
Syphilis (*Treponema pallidum* bacteria)	W&M: Disease has three stages: (1) single, painless sore, crater-like with smooth, rounded edges; (2) skin rash on back, stomach, hands, feet, flat,	Vaginal and anal intercourse. Oral-genital contact. Infected mother to newborn.	10 to 90 days; average 20 to 25 days.	Penicillin by injection; always have HIV test.	Serious for 30 percent who advance to stage 3; degeneration of major body systems, death;

(continued)

97

Table 5.2 (continued)

Infection/Cause	Symptoms	Transmission	Incubation Period	Treatments	Complications
	warty growths; and (3) severe damage to tissue, brain, and nervous system.				untreated pregnant women pass to newborn.
Trichomaniasis (*Trichomonas vaginalis* protozoa)	W: Vaginal discharge, burning, itching, odor. M: Penile discharge, burning, but rarely has symptoms.	Vaginal and anal intercourse.	About 7 days.	Oral antibiotics.	None serious.
Nongonococcal urethritis (NGU) (usually caused by chlamydia)	M: Same as chlamydia, gonorrhea.	Usually chlamydia.	7 to 21 days.	Oral antibiotics, treat partners, use condoms.	See chlamydia/gonorrhea.
Bacterial vaginosis (interaction of several bacteria)	W: Vaginal discharge, odor, itching, burning. M: No symptoms	Usually vaginal intercourse; however, BV can occur in women who abstain.	Unknown.	Oral antibiotics.	Seriousness unknown; may play role in postpartum infection/PID.

Note: W = women; M = men; W & M = women and men.
Source: Adapted from: http://www.birth-control-comparison.info/bc_pdf/sti_chart.pdf.

PROGRESSION OF HIV DISEASE

Initial Infection	Asymptomatic	Symptomatic	AIDS
1 to 3 months Antibodies can usually be detected during this time	Up to 10 years years or longer	May last 3 to 5 years or longer once they appear Chronic: Fever Diarrhea Swollen glands Weight loss Thrush Night sweats Fatigue Nausea	CD4 < 200 1 of 26 opportunistic infections, including Lymphomas Pulmonary Tuberculosis Pneumocystis Pneumonia Cytomegalovirus Herpes zoster Toxoplasmosis Kaposi's sarcoma Invasive cervical cancer Recurrent pneumonia

Source: Praeger, Sexual Health, 2007.

infected with HIV than are currently diagnosed (most of these people do not know they are infected).

Personal Account

I had a classmate in the 1990s who, when she tested positive for HIV, already had an AIDS diagnosis. She was a Caucasian woman in her early fifties who worked for a social service agency. She had kept getting sick with severe health issues, and her doctor tested her for multiple diseases and conditions trying to figure out what was wrong. I happened to be doing my internship at an AIDS organization at the time, and she talked to me at length one evening after class about symptoms of HIV. Shortly afterward, she asked her doctor, "What about HIV?" His response was that he did not think someone "like her" could be at risk. She then informed him that over 15 years prior, she had been an injection drug user. The doctor's bias and ignorance had kept her from an earlier diagnosis and treatment.

There tend to be certain groups of people at which society will point fingers in order to shirk responsibility for their own personal behaviors. I call this denial. HIV risk is not about who you are; it is about *what you do*. We are all sexual beings, and when we negotiate STI and HIV testing with a partner (if we even bother to do so), test negative, and choose to not use barriers for STIs, I do not call this safe sex. I call it a negotiated risk. I am not saying there is anything wrong with this, but even when we have established trust in the relationship through time and communication, life can happen. And for many people in sexual relationships, they have not discussed disease status or testing. Just something to consider.

Decreased Inhibitions

In terms of substance misuse and sexual risk, there are several connections to this spoke of the wheel. First of all, substance use can cloud judgment. Inhibitions are lowered when people are under the influence, and people may engage in behaviors that they normally wouldn't. It is not unusual for individuals to have sex with people they don't know or not use condoms when they are high. Motor judgment is also affected, and some people may use condoms incorrectly. There is also a risk for "blackouts." A blackout is when a person is under the influence, usually of alcohol, and functioning but with no memory of his or her behavior in a time period that can last from hours to days. I have literally heard stories from people where they "came out" of a blackout and were in bed with a stranger or in a place in which they had no recollection of how they got there. Blackouts are particularly dangerous, as a person could have had many behavioral risks (unprotected sex, being sexually assaulted, or sharing needles to inject drugs) but will have no memory of it. If the person is in a relationship, his or her partner may not be aware of the fact that the affected person is at any risk. In the event a person becomes infected with an STI during a blackout, for example, he or she may actually believe that his or her partner put him or her at risk or was the one who cheated because of this memory loss. So, drinking to the point of blackout is of particular concern for numerous reasons with regard to sexual risk.

Decreased Immune Function

Another, more indirect link to substance use is related to immune function. One of the functions of the liver is to produce white blood cells, which make up our immune system. The liver also filters out and processes toxins that pass through the body, so this includes any medications, drugs, and alcohol. When substances are being used, the liver's ability to produce normal amounts of white blood cells is decreased because of the increased load on the organ. A compromised immune system is more susceptible to infection and, if exposed to other diseases, such as HIV, several times more susceptible. So, if a person is under the influence, has sex, and is exposed to HIV, he or she has a greater chance of becoming infected.

STI and Substance Use as a Cofactor for HIV Transmission

Epidemiological evidence for STI as a cofactor for HIV transmission has emerged from several studies (Hayes & Schultz, 1992; Mortens, Hayes, & Smith, 1990; Pepin et al., 1989; Wasserheir, 1991). Separate from behavioral risk factors, both the ulcerative STIs (syphilis, chancroid, and genital herpes) and the discharge STIs (gonorrhea, chlamydia and trichomoniasis) are associated with increased risk of HIV transmission. The ulcerative STIs increase risk ninefold and the discharge diseases from three- to fivefold (Wasserheir, 1991).

A number of explanations can be offered to account for the role of STIs as cofactors in vaginal transmission of HIV infection: the breakdown of protective epithelial layers of skin and mucosal surfaces leading to exposure of blood vessels; elimination of protective, normal vaginal flora; alteration of the acidic pH of the vagina; and inflammation with the presence of CD4-positive target cells in the reproductive tract, to name a few (Hitchcock, 1996).

When a person has an STI, white blood cells (macrophages and B cells) flood the area affected in the process of creating an immune response and the production of antibodies. So, if a person is infected with a STI, the genital area contains high numbers of white blood cells. HIV infects the white blood cells, the presence of which during sexual activities creates a high-risk environment for coinfection with HIV if exposed. Untreated STIs create a high risk as well for similar reasons. Often, individuals are not aware of the presence of a STI and can be infected with one without showing symptoms. And if the uninfected person is not practicing safer sex and exposure to HIV occurs, he or she is at a much higher risk for coinfection with HIV.

Add alcohol or substance use, and the risk for actual infection is greatly enhanced. Undetected STI + HIV exposure + alcohol/substance use = high risk for infection. Given this brief analysis, it seems logical that prevention of STIs can assist in HIV prevention as well. Looking at the rates of STIs in the United States, it is increasingly apparent that there is a high infection rate that should not be ignored. Efforts to strengthen existing STI and HIV prevention programs and to develop new and creative ways to effectively control these treatable diseases could help in reducing new HIV infections. Finding creative methods to provide this programming in substance abuse treatment is vital to prevention efforts as well.

Injection Drug Use

Injecting substances is another risk for contracting STIs or HIV. Blood-borne pathogens, such as syphilis, hepatitis C, and HIV, are the most commonly transmitted infections through this route of ingestion. Of course, the main risk occurs when drug paraphernalia are shared or reused. If blood is present, then it poses a risk of transmitting bacteria or viruses. Indirect infection through injection drug use includes the sexual transmission of STIs or HIV from a primary partner to the sexual partner. A large number of women are infected from their partners' drug-using behaviors through sexual contact, or their babies can be indirectly infected through their past injection practices. Although risk of HIV infection from mother to infant can be greatly reduced through medications, knowledge of available protocols is necessary in order to properly educate clients.

USING A STAGING MODEL

Accurate and up-to-date information about HIV and STIs is critical to halt its spread. But, as many people knew all along, information is not enough (Prochaska, DiClemente, & Norcross, 1992). People need more than the facts—they need support in changing behaviors that put them at risk. Some effective strategies for HIV prevention are messages designed to teach people successful condom use strategies, such as how to negotiate condom use with partners who refuse to use condoms, attitudinal messages that clearly describe preventive outcomes of condom use, improving sexual communication, decreasing the number of sexual partners, and increasing both overall knowledge of and skills in applying prevention tactics (Johnson, Carey, Marsh, Levin, & Scott-Sheldon, 2003).

Utilizing a staging model based on the stages of change model can help us to stage our clients in sexual or other health behaviors. We talked about the process of behavior change through this lens previously. Asking the questions and using the model can help us to apply techniques appropriately. The following questions (remember RN-ACTS) can be used for assessing sexual behavior (or other) risk:

Step 1:

*R*elationship(s) in past three months

*N*umber of partners for client and client's partner(s)

- Identify target behavior—sexually inactive (SI), mutually monogamous uninfected partner (MMUP), safer sex (SS)

Step 2:

*A*ttitudes toward and history of the following:

*C*ondom use (male/female)

*T*esting (HIV status of client and client's partner[s])

- Assess client's stage of readiness to do target behavior

*S*ubstance Use

- Explore attitudes toward and history of substance use for client and client's partner(s)

(Center on Health and Behavioral Training, Rochester, New York)

The staging template (Table 5.3) can be used for any target behavior and illustrates how it can be used for staging clients in various health behaviors and attitudes along with the RN-ACTS tips. The overview of the transtheoretical model of change (Table 4.1 in Chapter 4) provides a brief reminder of counseling strategies matched to stages, and the sexual risk reduction grid (Table 5.4) is provided as an example for how to stage clients for reducing sexual risk of STI/HIV exposure.

HIV PREVENTION

The only sure way to prevent HIV infection is to avoid all contact with any body fluids that can transmit the virus (blood, semen, vaginal fluid, and breast milk). For sexual transmission, this means abstinence from all sexual behaviors that involve the exchange of blood semen or vaginal fluids, involvement in a mutually monogamous relationship with an uninfected partner, or the correct, consistent use of barrier methods that will prevent the passage of the virus from one person to another. Barrier methods are described in more detail at the end of this section.

Table 5.3   Staging Grid (fill in target behaviors for each client)

Stages of Change	Target Behavior	Target Behavior	Target Behavior
PC	PC Sees no need to . . .	PC Sees no need to . . .	PC Sees no need to . . .
C	C Sees need to, but . . .	C Sees need to, but . . .	C Sees need to, but . . .
RFA	RFA Ready to OR Has for less than 3 months	RFA Ready to OR Has for less than 3 months	RFA Ready to OR Has for less than 3 months
A	A Has consistently for 3–6 months	A Has consistently for 3–6 months	A Has consistently for 3–6 months
M	M Has consistently for greater than 6 months	M Has consistently for greater than 6 months	M Has consistently for greater than 6 months

Stages of Change:
PC: Precontemplative
C: Contemplative
RFA: Ready for action
A: Action
M: Maintenance

Target Behaviors:
*
*
*

Source: Adapted from the Center for Health and Behavioral Training, Rochester, New York.

For persons who inject substances, the following harm reduction approach is recommended, listed in hierarchal order from safest to least safe:

Safest: Abstinence (quit using altogether), including drug treatment as part of process.

Next safest: Methadone maintenance (for heroin) or buprenorphine. Methadone produces a high; buprenorphine reduces cravings and withdrawal, with no high.

Next safest: Find an alternative method of using; that is, snort or smoke the drug instead of injecting it.

Next safest: Don't share works (injection equipment). Each person has his or her own set of works.

Table 5.4   Staging Grid: Sexual Risk Reduction for HIV

Stages of Change	Sexually Inactive (SI)	Mutual Monogamy (MMUP)	Safer Sex (SS)
PC	PC, SI Not applicable	PC, MMUP Mutually monogamous for past 3 months, sees no need to test partner	PC, SS Multiple partners in past 3 months, sees no need to start using condoms consistently
C	C, SI Not applicable	C, MMUP Mutually monogamous for past 3 months, sees need to get partner tested, but . . .	C, SS Multiple partners in past 3 months, sees need to use condoms consistently, but . . .
RFA	RFA, SI Ready to stop having sex, OR Has not had sex for less than 3 months	RFA, MMUP Mutually monogamous for past 3 months, ready to get partner tested, OR With tested negative partner for less than 3 months	RFA, SS Multiple partners in past 3 months, ready to start using condoms consistently, OR Trying it for less than 3 months
A	A, SI Has not had sex for 3–6 months	A, MMUP Mutually monogamous with tested negative partner for 3–6 months	A, SS Multiple partners, using condoms consistently for 3–6 months
M	M, SI Has not had sex for greater than 6 months	M, MMUP Mutually monogamous with tested negative partner for greater than 6 months	M, SS Multiple partners, using condoms consistently for greater than 6 months

Stages of Change:
PC: Precontemplative
C: Contemplative
RFA: Ready for action
A: Action
M: Maintenance

Source: Adapted from the Center for Health and Behavioral Training, Rochester, New York.

Next safest: Use new needles every time for injection through a needle exchange program; in some states, a person can purchase syringes at a pharmacy without a prescription.

Next safest: Clean needles between sharing using the guidelines recommended by the CDC for cleaning:

3X 3X 3X method

1. Draw up clean water in syringe, shake for 30 seconds, and squirt out water (repeat two more times)
2. Draw up bleach in syringe, shake for 30 seconds, and squirt out bleach (repeat two more times)
3. Draw up clean water in syringe, shake for 30 seconds, and squirt out water (repeat two more times)

Next safest: Lesser steps and times in cleaning methods. Some people use bleach first, then water, and only rinse and squirt for 10 seconds once or twice. Anything is better than nothing.

Do not share cotton balls to stop bleeding, cookers to heat up drugs, ties to stop circulation, or anything that can pass blood from one person to another.

PREVENTING STIs

As was mentioned earlier, about half of all Americans will contract an STI at some point in their lifetime. With such a high incidence of infection, prevention of STIs is necessary to reduce risk behaviors and promote healthier lifestyles. Abstinence from sexual activity is the only 100 percent safe way to prevent acquiring an STI. Knowing your and your partner's personal sexual health status and negotiating a monogamous relationship is another way to reduce the risk of contracting an STI. For many people, however, it is stressful and embarrassing to discuss sexual matters, making disease prevention difficult to achieve. One study with 119 college couples found that most of the participants were unaware of their partners' past sexual experiences or risk behaviors (Seal, 1997).

The secrecy and shame associated with sexuality and STIs in particular make communication regarding sexual risk and past behaviors most embarrassing. But the truth of the matter is that if sexual partners are not comfortable in discussing sexual risk with one another, they are at high risk for exposure and infection. Learning strategies to initiate discussion with a potential sex partner is essential in preventing STIs and making smart sexual decisions. The following sections discuss basic guidelines for preventing exposure to STIs.

Know Your Sexual Health Status

If you are currently uninvolved in a sexual relationship, getting tested for STIs is an important step to take. It is possible that you may have an STI that you are unaware of, giving you the opportunity for treatment and secondary prevention or peace of mind knowing that you are disease free.

Assess a Potential Partner's Risk

Once you know your own sexual health status, think about getting to know a person before you become sexual with him or her. Often, people neglect to ask questions regarding past relationships or have a conversation about sexual matters. Some people will not be truthful when answering questions, but observing a person over a period of time may give you an indication of whether you feel you can trust that person. By taking the time to get to know someone, you may even be able to get tested together before initiating sexual activity. If the person is someone you have not taken time to get to know, then using protection would be the next step.

Use Barrier Methods with a Partner

This includes male and/or female condoms for vaginal and anal intercourse as well as condoms or barriers for oral intercourse. Condoms will prevent STIs when used correctly and consistently, but they are not 100 percent effective. For people who are new at using condoms, there can be a learning curve in using them correctly. If they are not used every time, they will be less effective. Some STIs, such as human papillomavirus or herpes simplex virus, can be on areas of the genitals where a condom does not cover, so if you or your partner has one of these viruses, it is important to be aware of whether and where your symptoms have occurred in order to reduce risk. In some instances, such as an outbreak of genital or oral herpes, abstaining from sexual activity or focusing on activities that do not involve the exchange of bodily fluids may be desirable.

Some persons have allergic reactions to latex; if this is the case, condoms made of polyurethane should be substituted. The female condom is made of polyurethane, as is the brand of male condoms Avanti. Using a condom that causes an allergic reaction can actually increase the risk of infection if exposed, as the skin can become irritated or develop a rash as a result.

When using condoms, the following guidelines should be considered as well:

- Always use a water-soluble lubricant (K-Y jelly or Astroglide) with condoms, as dry condoms can cause friction, and this can damage the mucous membranes, increasing risk.
- Never use oil-based lubricants with latex condoms. Latex is an oil-based product, and oil-based lubricants can cause the condom to break.
- Avoid using nonoxynol-9. Some condoms are lubricated with this spermicide, which may help prevent pregnancy, but it also can act as an irritant to the mucous membrane, which may actually increase risk of STIs.
- Check the packaging for expiration date and its condition. Outdated, worn-looking, brittle, or torn packaged condoms should be discarded.
- Take care when opening the package that nothing tears the condom, such as teeth or jewelry.
- Store condoms in a cool, dry place, out of direct sunlight. Try not to keep condoms in glove compartments of cars, wallets, or back pockets.
- Make sure you squeeze air out of the tip of the condom before it is rolled on. Air pockets can cause friction, weakening the condom. Roll the condom out over the erect penis; do not unroll the condom first and then try to put it on.
- Never use more than one condom: *no* double bagging. Two condoms can cause friction, weakening the condom. Latex condoms are petroleum-based products, and oil rubbing on oil can cause a blowout.
- If a condom does break, stop and replace it immediately.
- After ejaculation, hold the condom at the base when withdrawing to ensure that the condom does not slip off. Then take the condom off.
- Never reuse a condom.

Reduce or Avoid Sexual Activity with Multiple Partners

As discussed earlier, multiple sexual partners increase the risk for many STIs. Reducing or avoiding sexual activity with multiple partners will reduce a person's exposure to STIs. Persons with multiple sexual partners should have routine STI examinations in order to assess for infections even when no symptoms are present.

Inform a Partner If You Have an STI

This may seem like a formidable task, but if you find out that you have an STI while you are involved with another person, it is important that you inform him or her of your infection so that he or she can get treated and you do not continue to put each other at risk. The stigma associated with having an STI can make this conversation difficult, but it is healthier to have the discussion than to ignore it. Contracting an STI does not mean you are "bad" or "dirty." It simply means that you have an infection that needs attention, like any other health condition would. Because so many STIs do not produce obvious symptoms, it is a common occurrence to discover months or even years after the fact that you were infected with an STI.

Be honest in initiating the discussion. If you notice a discharge, bump, or sore, say so. Getting it checked out does not mean that you or your partner was unfaithful; you may have had the infection and not known about it. The way you approach the subject can influence how your partner may react. Choose a time when you are both relaxed. Do not blame the other person; nothing will be gained from this approach. If you take an up-front, matter-of-fact tone, you may be able to resolve the matter in a caring way.

Try to be sensitive to your partner's feelings and reactions. It is understandable for someone to be angry or upset at this type of news. Being supportive and not reacting defensively to them may help you work through initial responses. Think about how you would feel if it were your partner telling you the same news.

In some instances, the local health department or health care providers can do partner notification. Some benefits of utilizing health department notification is that the person being notified will receive counseling to reduce further risk of exposure, treatment, and testing options. Utilizing these services is beneficial when notifying past sexual partners is not practical for the infected person. Partner notification is crucial to treat infected persons and to curtail the spread of infections.

SAMPLE LESSONS FOR HIV AND SAFER SEX

Values Activity

Goal: To assist participants in examining values and attitudes they hold toward HIV/AIDS and other sexual risk behaviors and help them to understand the relationship between their attitudes and related substance use.
Rationale: By examining values and attitudes related to sexual behaviors and HIV/AIDS, participants can consider how the impact of those beliefs

shape their behaviors in relation to maintaining abstinence from drugs and alcohol. For example, a woman may have a belief that casual sex is wrong but has frequently engaged in sexual encounters, trading sexual favors for drugs. During a treatment attempt, she got tested for HIV, tested positive, and left treatment prematurely. She never dealt with the inner conflict and continued to use chemicals to numb out her feelings. This conflict may not be easily resolved unless she reexamines her beliefs and modifies them in order to deal with the resulting shame and trauma. This particular type of activity would ideally follow a session on HIV/STI information.

Time: 90 minutes
Objectives: Participants will do the following:

- Identify some of the attitudes and values one holds about HIV/AIDS
- Examine and discuss the impact HIV/AIDS may have on their lives and the recovery process
- Identify personal attitudes and values about sexual risk and drug-using behaviors
- Examine and discuss the impact sexual risk and drug-using behaviors may have had on their lives and the recovery process

Materials:

- Signs on 8½-by-11 paper—"A great deal," "Not at all"
- Continuum signs on 8½-by-11 paper—"Strongly agree," "Agree," "Not sure," "Disagree," and "Strongly disagree"
- Enough handouts of values clarification exercise (Appendix C)
- Sexual Beingness sheets

Values Clarification: (40 minutes)
Place the continuum signs across a wall in order from "Strongly disagree" to "Strongly agree." Distribute the values clarification sheets and ask participants to rate their values for each statement. Assist anyone who needs help reading. After about five minutes, ask them to stand under the attitude with which they most identify when you read selected statements. The facilitator should choose four or five statements that relate most to the desired outcomes of the activity (values statements can be adapted for use in other groups, depending on topic).

After each selected value statement is read and participants go to their placement, ask each person to provide a reason for the response he or she chose. There should be no discussion, just a verbal response that gets heard by the group without interruption. Read the next value statement and repeat the process.

When the selected value statements are all read, use the following process questions to facilitate a large-group discussion:

1. How did it feel to speak about your value in front of others?
2. How did it feel when one of your values was one of the minority opinions?
3. What was it like to not be able to respond to others statements?
4. In what ways did some of the responses affect how you felt about yourself?
5. In what ways are your feelings connected to any of your substance-using behaviors?

The facilitator should process a discussion around issues that are raised concerning topical matters in the activity. Depending on any questions or disagreements that may ensue based on specific value statements, clarification of information and allowing differing points of views to be shared may be warranted.

Examining values in sexual health education is critical to affecting attitudes and lasting behavior change. If sexuality education is taught from one viewpoint, without challenging learners to examine their beliefs and have the opportunity to obtain information from multiple views, we limit the options and abilities of individuals to make informed or healthy choices that make sense to them. If controversial subjects are taught, then a range of viewpoints must be discussed and reviewed in the context of a rational, democratic philosophy (Gilgun & Gordon, 1983). Information and group discussion will involve participants to discuss a variety of views and options.

Values clarification is included for participants to reexamine the reasons they hold certain views and opinions as well as to listen to how others view similar issues. We can't facilitate effective behavior change unless we get to why people hold the beliefs they do. People won't change their thinking unless it makes sense to them, and processing the activity to discuss why people believe what they do allows others to consider viewpoints that are different then their own, allowing for the possibility of a modified belief as a result. Finally, addressing shaming messages internalized from others values is critical in the process of helping validate the experiences.

The discussion that follows each activity is a critical component of effective learning. Constructing process questions that probe the sensitive nature of people's feelings will stimulate a challenging and meaningful group experience. Participants are encouraged to respond to comments and questions posed by the facilitator and other group members in order to facilitate critical thinking skills and thought in regard to the material. Discussion is encouraged to help build participants' confidence in their personal value to the group. Facilitators need to provide supportive feedback in order to reward discussion among the group members.

How Has HIV/AIDS Affected You? (40 minutes)
Place the continuum signs on opposite sides of the room and ask participants to stand on an imaginary line for each of the following after making this statement: "How has HIV affected you?" (For the extreme of each statement, i.e., if the statement had moderate affect, participants may be in the middle of the room between both signs). Do each one, one at a time:

• Personally
• In an intimate relationship
• In the way you negotiate a new relationship

After participants line themselves up on how HIV has affected them, have them share (to the extent they are comfortable and you have time) how they have been impacted. Some who may not see how they have been impacted may change their positions after hearing from others. You may want to suggest they can change positions at any time. This can be a very powerful exercise and rich discussion after each of the continuum placements.

Break them into small groups and have them discuss how HIV/AIDS affects our culture and themselves in relation to the following:

• Abstinence
• Monogamy
• Lesbian/gay/bisexuality
• Casual sex
• Condom use
• Drug and alcohol use

Bring the group together after about 10 minutes and use the following process questions to facilitate a large-group discussion:

1. How does it feel to talk about this?

2. What are some of your observations about the discussion, and what you were thinking/feeling?

3. What did you learn that might help you in your recovery process?

After group process, distribute the Sexual Beingness sheets and ask participants to circle any items on the sheet that they felt were addressed in the session as well as to write on the back of the sheet a couple of things that they learned about themselves from the session.

CREATING YOUR WORK OF ART

Presenting information to client groups is critical for facilitating positive behavior change and promoting sexual health. When using the stages of change model, we need to stage our client group in order to choose the best approach. Is the group precontemplative? If so, providing information may help move them into contemplation. Are they contemplative? If so, providing activities that ask them to consider their personal risk with the issue or examining their attitudes or values may facilitate some movement toward taking action. I always try to take into account the characteristics of my group whenever possible. If you do not know your group, a mix of activities can ensure that your program will appeal to most of the group members at some level. If this is a client group that you work with on a regular basis, you have the luxury of planning activities that will enhance your group's experience. Of course, successful group facilitation is an art, learned over time. I want you all to be Rembrandts.

RESOURCES

Books

Berkowitz, R. (2003). *Stayin' alive: The invention of safe sex*. Boulder, CO: Westview Press.

Joannides, P. (2011). *The guide to getting it on*. Waldport, OR: Goofy Foot Press.

Online Resources

AIDSinfo. http://www.aidsinfo.nih.gov.

CDC. http://www.cdc.gov/nchstp/dstd/disease_info.htm.

Medline Plus. http://www.nlm.nih.gov/medlineplus/sexuallytransmitted diseases.html.

Sex Smart Films. http://www.sexsmartfilms.com.

SIX

Sensitive Issues and Challenges

You know what? It just sucks. But we'll get through it.

—Shannon, Welcome to Barbados, http://www.pandys.org/escaping hades/quotations.html

We expect teachers to handle teenage pregnancy, substance abuse, and the failings of the family. Then we expect them to educate our children.

—John Sculley

A lot of people in our community don't want to believe that child abuse happens in their neighborhoods—but it does.

—Shari Pulliam, http://www.allgreatquotes.com/child_abuse_sex _abuse_quotes.shtml

Any topic can be sensitive, depending on what is personal to individuals; keeping this in mind when discussing certain topics is helpful to know. This is also another reason to incorporate attitudinal activities in group work because eliciting strong emotional reactions to selected topics can assist counselors in identifying potential relapse triggers in their clients. There are many challenges to consider when working with addicted individuals in the treatment setting. With regard to sexuality, some of these include the following:

- Sexual, physical, and/or emotional abuse or assault
- Rape, incest, or molestation
- Sexual dysfunction

- Infection with HIV/sexually transmitted diseases
- Reproductive issues, such as infertility, unwanted pregnancy, and abortion
- Sexual harassment
- Out-of-control sexual behavior
- Sexual orientation issues
- Gender identity
- Sexism
- Intimacy

Discussing these topics in treatment can be intimidating for both the client and the counselor. There has been the belief by many providers that by broaching these "sensitive" areas, the proverbial Pandora's box will be opened and clients immediately relapse or self-destruct. This myth is far from the truth. In fact, by avoiding sexual issues, we are doing a disservice to clients by not opening the door to areas that can benefit from exploration and open discussion. If part of the reason I drink every day has to do with the incest I suffered by a family member, then how am I to recover if I cannot process the connections to my use patterns and devise a recovery plan for when and if I will be faced with my perpetrator at future family gatherings? Avoidance of sexual issues on the part of providers is due in part to their own personal discomfort with sexuality issues and lack of knowledge of what to say. As there is considerable overlap in other chapters regarding some of the previously listed challenges, sexual abuse/assault, rape, molestation, incest, and out-of-control sexual behavior are the main challenges addressed in this section.

SEXUAL ABUSE, RAPE, MOLESTATION, AND INCEST

Which comes first, the chicken or the egg? This question is often asked when exploring variables related to substance misuse. Sexual abuse issues can make one vulnerable to the use and misuse of substances, and substance use in and of itself can lead to exposure to abusive and sexual risk situations. When examining the etiology of substance use, causation is often linked to multiple areas, including environment, culture, genetics, temperament, associative memory, and more. Identifying the relevant correlations is the first step.

Research on sexual and physical abuse suggests that individuals with such histories are more likely to report higher levels of alcohol consumption. Both men and women with sexual or physical abuse histories report a higher level of general psychological distress than do their nonabused counterparts (Bryer, Nelson, Miller, & Krol, 1987; Swett, Surrey, & Cohen, 1990). Survivors of trauma are reportedly more likely to have anxiety and depression (Grice,

Brady, Dustan, Malcom, & Kilpatrick, 1995; Wilsnack, Vogeltanz, Klassen, & Harris, 1997) as well as personality disorders (Grice et al., 1995). Victims of sexual and physical abuse (Brown & Finkelhor, 1986) exhibit poor interpersonal relationship functioning. In a sample of inpatient alcoholics, Windle, Windle, Schedit, and Miller (1995) found that both sexual abuse and combined sexual and physical abuse—but not physical abuse only—were associated with generalized anxiety disorder and antisocial personality.

CO-OCCURRING DISORDERS

Common psychiatric diagnoses that can result in part from past sexual abuse include borderline personality disorder, eating disorders, dissociative disorders, and addictive disorders (Berliner & Elliot, 1996). Child sexual abuse survivors are also likely to develop posttraumatic stress disorder symptoms. If the abuse involved force or penetration was present, the likelihood of developing the disorder is high (Heffernan & Cloitre, 2000; Kendall-Tackett, Williams, & Finkelhor, 1993). Survivors of childhood sexual abuse have a posttraumatic stress disorder prevalence rate of almost 50 percent (Kendall-Tackett et al., 1993). In general, symptoms of sexual abuse vary; in fact, up to 50 percent of children who have been sexually abused may exhibit no symptoms (Hansen, Hecht, & Futa, 1998). A large meta-analysis (a study that examines dozens of research studies) of sexual abuse research found that sexual abuse may not always result in negative consequences, depending on the circumstances surrounding the abuse (Rind & Tromovitch, 1997).

SEVERITY OF ABUSE

Abuse involving penetration, multiple offenders, violence, and more frequent occurrences, as well as a closer relationship with the perpetrator, appear to result in a greater psychological and behavioral impact (Kendall-Tackett et al., 1993). Similarly, abuse that involved some form of penetration was more likely to result in more symptoms than abuse that did not. The identity of the perpetrator was found to be directly related to the severity of impact, usually fathers or stepfathers, resulting in greater impact on a child.

UNDERSTANDING LINKS

Understanding the links and their connections can assist providers in identifying triggers for clients, helping to develop appropriate referrals and treatment plans as well as providing insight into the unique circumstances that contribute to the addiction process. By taking the time to assess and evaluate a sexual history that includes challenges and sensitive issues, counselors can provide new avenues for recovery to their clientele. Having the conversations at multiple times opens the door for permission to discuss sexual issues. Every time I have gone into agencies to facilitate focus groups or run sexuality programming, clients express their relief to me in being able to discuss sexuality-related issues. Many claim that no one at the agency has broached sexual topics. A few agencies do provide groups, usually trauma based, that include some sexuality issues but not comprehensively. I propose that a sexual health group that is run concurrently with trauma-informed treatment can provide a stronger foundation for improved treatment outcomes.

ASSESSMENT AND DEFINING ABUSE

One of the first issues to consider in identifying sexual health challenges is assessment. Any researcher can attest to the importance of how we ask questions to obtain our data. And in the case of sensitive issues, knowing what to ask as well as how and when to ask it can be critical to obtaining honest and accurate information from our clients. Abuse can be defined differently by people, depending on one's beliefs and values regarding what constitutes abuse, so using language that elicits specific behaviors can be helpful. In terms of assessing for physical, sexual, and emotional abuse, the abuse questionnaire has been used in several of my research studies with good outcomes.

General identification of sexual issues is sufficient for choosing activities in a sexual health group with regard to exploration of abuse. This assessment elicits very general information that is nonthreatening to clients and gently opens that door. Often, the details surrounding abuse come out in groups or individual counseling once there is a venue for discussion. It is important to let clients describe their own personal experiences rather than impose detailed questionnaires that may overwhelm them.

Defining Abuse

In terms of defining sexual abuse, sexual abuse involves any sexual activity, including unwanted touch where consent either is not or cannot be given. Child sexual abuse involves any sexual activity with a child where consent either is not or cannot be given (Finkelhor, 1979). This includes sexual contact that is accomplished by force or threat of force, regardless of age. All sexual contact between an adult and a child, regardless of the child's understanding of the nature of the activity is considered sexual abuse (Berliner & Elliot, 1996). There are a variety of behaviors and activities that constitute sexual abuse, including sexual penetration, touching, and noncontact sexual acts, such as exposure or voyeurism. Incest is child sexual abuse that occurs between family members, including blood relatives, stepparents, in-laws, and extended family (Finkelhor, 1979).

ABUSE QUESTIONNAIRE

The term "partner" is used to describe any person you consider to be (or have been) in an intimate relationship with, regardless of gender. Ideally, relationships are loving and supportive, protective of, and safe for each member of the couple. Unfortunately, some people, while fulfilling these nurturing and positive needs of their partners at least some of the time and at least early on in their relationship's development, also behave abusively, causing their partners (and often other as well) substantial emotional, physical, and sexual abuse. This survey is intended to help us determine whether or not you have been a victim of emotional, physical and/or sexual abuse.

Please place a check mark next to each question that applies to your experience.

1. _____ Have you ever been smacked, beaten, kicked, choked, or in any other way physically abused in the course of your life?

2. _____ Have you ever been physically abused by any other important person in your life (for example, parent, relative)?

3. _____ Have you ever been physically abused by your partner?

4. _____ Are you afraid of anyone in your family or surroundings who may physically abuse you?

5. _____ Has anyone ever pressured you into sexual activities when your did not want them to?

6. _____ Has anyone ever touched you in a way that you did not want them to?

7. _____ Have you ever been forced to perform sexual activity by another person?

8. _____ Are you afraid of anyone in your family of physical surroundings who may sexually abuse you?

9. _____ Has your partner ever said mean or hurtful things to you?

10. _____ Has your partner ever done any of the following:
    - Criticized you in front of others
    - Restricted your behavior in some way
    - Told you that you were inferior
    - Brought up past relationships with the intent to hurt you
    - Threatened to leave you
    - Threatened to harm you

> - Destroyed your belongings
> - Harmed a pet or your children (or threatened to)
>
> If you answered yes, to any of the above, was the experience:
> Past _____Present_____Both _____
> How would you describe the person involved:
> Parent_____Family Member _____Stranger _____Partner _____
> Other (specify):_____
> How old were you when this occurred? _____
>
> *Source*: Adapted from Parker and McFarlane (1991).

Client Experiences

In all of my research thus far with women in treatment for substance abuse, over 90 percent of participants self-reported combinations of sexual, physical, and/or emotional abuse. Abuse also took many forms, including rape, sexual assault, and incest. Take, for example, the case of one young African American woman:

> I been using drugs since I was nine years old. I started smoking pot with my grandfather. I also suffered incest at the hands of my own father. I was very promiscuous with members of my family, um, my father, and my grandfather, my uncles, and my cousins, um, and I thought that that was normal and that was natural to be sleeping around with members of the people in my family. I didn't really sleep around with or engage in any activities with outside people, just amongst my family members who I was promiscuous with.

This particular woman also had experiences of rape that she shared with the group. The effect of her disclosure was very powerful and enabled many of the other women to open up about similar abuse situations:

> I am HIV positive, and that has what caused me to relapse this last time around. I do shoot heroin, but I was HIV positive due to the fact that I was raped in every hole in my body. I'm an ex-prostitute; the guy left me for dead, and he infected me with this virus. I found out that I was infected during the pregnancy. I went for my prenatal care with my daughter, and they told me that I was HIV positive, and I definitely wanted to commit suicide. I wanted to die, um, I didn't know

if my baby was going to live, I didn't understand, but now I've got a great strong support system. I go to support groups; that is why I'm still alive. I go to the doctor pretty regularly; my parents know, my family knows, they don't treat me any different, they love me still unconditionally, uh, and I have been learning to love myself and just accept that fact that I am not a victim, that I am a survivor of a lot of different abuse and trauma that's gone on in my life.

This particular woman had not yet disclosed her HIV status in treatment, so for her to self-disclose in a focus group being run by outside researchers speaks in part to the sensitivity utilized in our facilitation of the group. She felt safe enough, in a very short time frame (during introductions in fact), to share very personal information regarding her experiences with us. Needless to say, having this information about a client in treatment would be critical to address in terms of treatment planning regarding the incest, feelings of shame, struggles with HIV status, guilt over potential perinatal transmission (she did not mention her daughter's age or HIV status in the group), effects of trauma, and connections to substance use. I could spend a great deal of time working this into treatment planning, identifying with her which issues were pressing (or not) and also with relapse prevention and aftercare plans. By not having this information, providers miss an opportunity to identify numerous issues related to sexuality, addiction, and recovery. I often hear people use the phrase "what we don't know, won't hurt us." Nothing could be further from the truth.

Gender Differences

Females have a tendency to internalize their traumatizing symptom effects by showing more signs of anxiety, fear, and depression (Finkelhor, Hotaling, Lewis, & Smith, 1990; Kendall-Tackett et al., 1993; Spacarrelli, 1994). Alternatively, males seem to have a tendency to cope with their abuse by externalizing their distress, often displaying aggression and anger. They tend to manifest their anxiety through sexual and physical aggressiveness (Scott, 1992). Additionally, boys may have a heightened preoccupation with sexual activity, a generalized attitude of hypermasculinity (aggressiveness, explosions of temper, and discouraged expression of vulnerability) and extreme fear of homosexuality. This homophobia makes boys rigid in expression of typical male characteristics (i.e., machismo) and instills a fear of close relationships with other males.

Male victims often perceive themselves as emotionally and physically weak for being the object of abuse (Scott, 1992; Zamanian & Adams, 1997). These authors assert that male victims will display aggression, a hypermasculine stance, and sexual identity confusion and may have a compulsion to repeat their experiences in a masochistic or sadistic way. In terms of the relationship of male victimization and externalized expression, the high occurrences of perpetrators were reportedly men (Scott, 1992). In fact, nearly 96 percent of perpetrators whose victims were males are men (Reinhart, 1987). Some believe that this victim/victimizer pattern is a means of protection so as not to be revictimized.

In terms of gender differences, research suggests that there are more similarities than differences between male and female survivors of child sexual abuse. However, there are several differences that deserve mention. Predominantly male concerns include the following:

- They are more often abused by teachers, coaches, and babysitters.
- As a result of child sexual abuse at the hand of a male offender, males struggle with their sexual identity and fears of homosexuality. Men who experienced child sexual abuse find it harder to define their gender roles.
- Both male victims and their parents are more likely to try to minimize the impact of the sexual abuse.
- Male survivors are more likely to abuse drugs.
- Boys are more likely to be sodomized than girls.
- Men are more likely to experience anger and rage in the early stages of recovery, whereas their feelings of grief tend to surface later in the healing process. Men have more struggles with feelings of powerlessness, and the chances of active and violent revenge fantasies are greater.
- Far fewer men than women consider their early childhood sexual experiences to be sexual abuse. Gender socialization, different physiological responses of the sexes, and culturally determined expressions of sexuality may cause boys to be neutral or positive about their sexual experiences, but the long-term effects (e.g., on self-esteem) are negative.
- Male survivors carry a stigma because male victims may often feel responsible when things go wrong; this is a belief perpetuated by societal expectations that males ought to be in control of their sexual encounters and able to take care of themselves (Women's Web, 2011).

Predominantly female concerns include the following:

- Female survivors are at greater risk for abusing alcohol.
- There is a greater chance that the abuse will take place in the home and be perpetrated by somebody related to the victim.

- Female survivors are at greater risk of being revictimized as teenagers and young adults.
- They are more likely to receive support when dealing with their recovery issues.
- Compared with men, women tend to deal with their sadness and depression in the early stages of recovery, whereas their anger seems to surface later in the healing process.
- Women appear to have greater difficulty in recalling specific details connected to the abusive situation.
- Among victims of child sexual abuse, girls are fondled more often than boys.
- Female survivors often carry more stigma than male survivors; female survivors are often blamed in whole or in part for their abuse. Others' responses to a female's abuse and their judgments can become an intrinsic part of the woman's own beliefs about what happened to her; they can have a serious impact on her self-image (Women's Web, 2011).

In comparing the experiences of male and female survivors, it's important to avoid using "more" or "less" since the experience of being abused cannot be quantified and should not be the subject of value judgments. Ultimately, the perceived experience of being abused lies with the survivor.

When facilitating sexuality groups in the treatment process, I recommend strongly that groups be separated by gender for several reasons. First, many women have been victimized and/or sexually traumatized by men, and by mixing genders in a treatment group, women may not feel safe to explore these issues. Second, as men's issues take different trajectories, men may feel threatened exploring sexual abuse issues in a mixed group for fear of "losing face" or not appearing traditionally masculine around women. They will often put on the tough guise of being macho as a front and to keep up a wall for not showing vulnerability. Last but not least, by keeping groups gender specific, each gender can also work through trust issues with their respective gender, as many men and women have not learned how to develop positive relationships with people of the same sex as well. Counselors should take this consideration to heart and have the ability to be cognizant of gender differences and be able to recognize any gender issues present with the sex of their participants. In fact, cofacilitating sexuality groups with both female and male group leaders can set a positive tone as well. By having sensitivity to and knowledge of women's and men's issues, facilitators can be a powerful force in this recovery process.

Effects of Abuse on Clients

Effects may take different forms at different stages of a survivor's life and recovery. Occasionally, the effects of having been sexually abused can remain guarded or "hidden away"—repression and dissociation are protective mechanisms often used by survivors to keep the memory of their abuse out of their consciousness. Although on the surface these coping mechanisms may appear to shield survivors, over the long term they may prove harmful because they keep survivors from dealing with their pain and trauma—pain and hurt that can resurface again or be triggered by significant life events.

In the course of a person's life, being victimized by sexual abuse or assault may not have ever been discussed. Reasons for this include having been threatened at the time by the perpetrator, and if the event(s) took place at an early age, internalized fear of telling may have prevented subsequent disclosure. Other common reactions of family members on hearing of abuse (in particular, incest) are feelings of disbelief and denial. For victims sharing the abuse for the first time, this type of response can effectively shut them down emotionally again and serve as a form of revictimization, especially if the perpetrators had told them they would not be believed if they ever told:

Casey: I feel like that, um, because of the sexual abuse as a child, once I learned because as a child I thought it was okay. Once I got older and learned that it wasn't, and I didn't tell anyone until I was 14 years old. And it happened from the time til I was 5 til I was 9, and, um, when I did tell, they didn't believe me. And, uh, so I felt kind of like an outcast. I started using a little before 14. But at 14 after all that happened and I felt like my family pushed me away because of it. I thought I was just a problem child or you know I wanted attention or something. I don't actually know what they actually thought, but that's how I felt. And my substance abuse got more, it got heavier after that. And I started running away from home a lot, and then I was involved in the court system, and then I was in foster homes, and then it started happening again. And I felt like if I told anybody, that they wouldn't believe me, and I drank a lot when I was younger. And I would drink until I just could not stand up or function or anything, and I just, I feel like it was because I didn't want to; I felt bad, I felt dirty, I felt, um, abandoned I guess, there were a lot of different things going on, but I think that now that I've learned a little more about it, I think that that had a lot to do with it.

Maria: In the Latina culture, especially the older generations, they tend to accuse you instead of helping you. Blame you for the sexual abuse or the incest or whatever. Or keep in the house and don't, you know, what happens at home you should be ashamed of. . . . Most of the time they just plain out don't believe you, and the other family members, some of them will hear it and then turn around and molest you too.

These clients (and many more) expressed deep connections to feelings of shame associated with their experiences of not being believed or being blamed for the abuse and incest. Many factors can impact a survivor's response to his or her abuse, including the following:

- Being believed
- Personal resources
- Availability of emotional support
- Access to financial resources to pay for treatment
- Time between abuse and the start of treatment or psychotherapy
- Cultural/ethnicity factors
- Current or chronic life stressors
- Age and maturity of the victim
- Response of family members or significant others
- Prior knowledge about sex and sexuality
- The degree to which the victim felt that he or she had some control over what happened
- Reframing his or her negative experiences in a positive way
- Access to supportive relationships with other adults or significant others
- Hope and an optimistic outlook on the future
- Being given skills to avoid future risky situations (Women's Web, 2011)

COMMON BELIEFS ABOUT ABUSE

Erroneous information about sexual abuse/assault is important to dispel so that providers do not let false beliefs cloud the work they do with clients. The following is a brief description of some common beliefs regarding abuse issues and information that may in turn help providers to normalize their clients' experiences. For example, the previous client experiences of being accused of lying or fantasizing about sexual activities with adults can be countered with accurate information and validate the abuse scenarios that were shared in the group. After one of our sessions, a client verbalized relief in being believed and told by us that the abuse was not her fault. This helped to move her forward in the recovery process.

I often hear people say that children lie about sexual abuse. Young children are not cognitively able to conceive what sexual abuse is unless it has happened to them. Often, if they do lie, it is to protect the person who has abused them out of fear or having been threatened. Perpetrators often threaten their older child victims with bodily harm, abuse of a sibling or family member, or worse.

The secrecy surrounding incest is a particularly damaging phenomenon, as revealed in several of my client interviews. Victims of incest are often extremely reluctant to reveal that they are being abused because their abuser is a person in a position of trust and authority for the victim. Often incest victims do not understand (or they deny) that anything is wrong with the behavior they are encountering (Vanderbilt, 1992). Many young incest victims accept and believe the perpetrator's explanation that this is a "learning experience" that happens in every family by an older family member. Incest victims may fear they will be disbelieved, blamed, or punished if they report their abuse. Some believe or are coerced to believe that the family will break up if they tell and that the responsibility lies with the child.

Sexual abuse in families is not typically a one-time incident. For most victims, the abuse continues for years. Offenders do not usually stop unless they are caught or there is an intervention (Spelman, 1993).

Nonviolent sexual abuse can also be traumatizing, depending on the age and way in which the abuse is perpetrated. Abuse in the form of sexual harassment, such as unwanted touch, unwelcome sexual advances, requests for sexual favors, and verbal or physical contact of a sexual nature, can be extremely damaging and intimidating. Children are more vulnerable because of their lack of power and status. Adults, particularly in work environments, may experience great anxiety and stress-related effects. Imagine going to work every day knowing that someone will harass you, make sexual jokes, request sexual favors, and stare at your body every chance they get. A hostile workplace can be threatening indeed.

Many people think that men and boys cannot be sexually abused, assaulted, or raped. If "you were a real man," you could be masculine enough to fight off an attacker. In U.S. culture, there is a belief that male + masculine = heterosexual. Being a male victim of rape is inherently viewed as a feminine act: only women get raped because they are weak and vulnerable. So, it goes to say that men and boys who are raped and sexually assaulted must be gay, or why would they have attracted this type of assault? Nothing could be further from the truth, but, unfortunately, this type of thinking permeates the consciousness as a result of a heterosexist society.

Another belief is that children provoke sexual abuse by their seductive behavior. Often, seductive behavior can result from being sexually abused, as young girls and women learn that they get the attention of men through flirting and acting sexual. Behavior considered by many to be seductive and promiscuous is typically a result of prior abuse. Regardless of the victim's behavior or reason for such behavior, the responsibility for appropriate behavior always lies with the adult, not the child. A teenage girl is no match for the manipulative tactics of a man twice her age; therefore, the ability to affect adult consent is unreasonable to expect (Neddermeyer, 2011). Often adolescents who are displaying seductive behavior are not developmentally prepared to comprehend the etiology and consequences of their actions.

If the victim experiences sexual arousal or orgasm from abuse, they are perceived as having been a willing participant or having enjoyed it. Physiological arousal to genital stimulation (vaginal lubrication or erections) is an automatic response, triggered by touch. This does not equate to enjoyment or pleasure. Sometimes perpetrators manipulate their victims into secrecy, utilizing shame and guilt as a weapon as a result of the sexual arousal response. Physical, visual, or auditory stimulation is likely to occur in a sexual situation. It does not mean that the child wanted the experience or understood what it meant (Neddermeyer, 2011).

Another belief is that the effects of sexual abuse are permanent. Depending on the age of the victim, the severity of the abuse, whether it was kept a secret, and whether the person was believed and supported after disclosing can all impact a recovery trajectory. Typically, time, counseling, and support will help people heal from the effects of sexual abuse (Brown & Finkelhor, 1986). Although memories and psychological and physical reactions may be triggered by touch, smells, sexual activity, or exposure to movies with sexual content, these negative responses can learn to be controlled and reduced in severity and frequency with the aid of cognitive-behavioral interventions and other therapeutic techniques (Hansen et al., 1998).

Talking about sexual abuse with children is not damaging; inaccurate or no information can be more damaging. It is important for children to receive information about sexual abuse and assault not only for preventive measures but also to intervene if abuse is suspected or confirmed. The longer a caregiver waits to provide supportive action, the more damage is incurred, especially with incest and child abuse (Bass & Davis, 1988; Spelman, 1993; Vanderbilt, 1992).

TRAUMAGENIC DYNAMICS MODEL OF SEXUAL ABUSE

Finkelhor & Browne (1985) have described a traumagenic dynamics model of sexual abuse to explain the unique factors associated with the experience of childhood sexual abuse. The model acknowledges the different effects of child sexual abuse, depending on the nature of the abuse, while specifying its impact on a child's development. The model consisted of four key experiences that alter a child's cognitive or emotional orientation to the world and distort the child's self-concept, view of others, and affective functioning (Finkelhor & Browne, 1985; Spacarrelli, 1994).

The first experience is called traumatic sexualization. This involves exposure to sexual experiences that are developmentally inappropriate. Traumatic sexualization is thought to increase sexual acting out, confusion regarding sexual identity, and compulsive sexuality or sexual aversion (Finkelhor & Browne, 1985).

Powerlessness, the second experience in Finkelhor & Brownes (1985) model, denotes the inability of the child to stop or prevent the abuse. This experience is thought to cause anxiety and a tendency to see oneself as a victim in a multitude of situations and may lead to identification with the perpetrator. Some behavioral outcomes of this experience are somatic complaints, depression, dissociation, sexually aggressive behavior, and phobias (Finkelhor & Browne, 1985).

Stigmatization, the third experience, occurs when negative connotations of the experience are communicated to the child. This is thought to lower self-esteem and cause feelings of shame and guilt. Stigmatization often leads to substance abuse, social isolation, suicidality, and self-harm behaviors (Finkelhor & Browne, 1985).

Realization that a trusted person has manipulated or failed to protect the child is the fourth and final experience explained in the model. This experience of betrayal shatters the child's confidence that trusted people are capable of protecting him or her. When experiencing this stage of the model, children often exhibit clingy behavior. They additionally display conduct problems, mistrust, grief, and anger (Finkelhor & Browne, 1985).

We should never generalize abuse characteristics across the board, as there are many variations in client responses to abuse. Exploring these variations in treatment will enable providers to provide appropriate intervention, referrals, and support. Utilization of group therapy, eye movement desensitization and reprocessing, processing of feelings regarding abuse and perpetrators, sex education, prevention, and identification of support systems are some recommended techniques and approaches for sexually abused clients (Berliner & Elliot, 1996; Hack, Osachuk, & DeLuca, 1994; Sirles, Walsma, Lytle-Barnaby, & Lander, 1988).

OUT-OF-CONTROL SEXUAL BEHAVIOR

This area of our sexual health model concerns sexual behaviors that can be linked to substance abuse in problematic ways. The use of the terms "sexual addiction" and "out-of-control sexual behavior" have been used to describe this phenomenon to various degrees in several professional fields, including the addiction field. Within psychology, there tends not to be agreement over whether excessive sexual behavior can be described as an addictive disorder, an impulsive behavior, an obsessive-compulsive behavior, or a psychosexual disorder. Definitions are commonly conceptualized by those in sexual health to be "the uncontrolled tendency to engage in sex-related activities in a persistent manner despite possible negative consequences to self and to others" (Perera, Reece, Monahan, Billingham, & Finn, 2009, p. 88).

COMPETING VIEWS OF SEXUALITY

Historically in the United States, the concept of "controlled" and "uncontrolled" sexual behaviors has been used to argue against the notion of sexual deviancy (Braun-Harvey, 1997). "What one society regards as being sexually out of control or deviant may or may not be viewed as such in another" (Levine & Troiden, 1988, p. 351). Three normative but competing views of sexual behavior currently exist in the United States, namely, procreational, relational, or recreational:

This means that for some, sexual pleasure can be valued only when limited to the context of procreation within a heterosexual marriage. For others, sexual contact can also be a means of expressing and reinforcing one's emotional and psychological intimacy within any committed relationship. Still others view erotic feelings and sexual expressions between mutually consenting adults, even between strangers, without emotional commitment as acceptable behaviors. These conflicting views create an underlying tension in the conceptualization and treatment of sexual dependency. (Braun-Harvey, 1997, p. 362)

Misdiagnosing

On the basis of this premise and in the event that past sexual behavior is documented as negative or damaging to an individual's personal/professional existence, a diagnosis or label of sexual compulsivity or sexual addiction is generally given to a client in substance abuse treatment (Irvine, 1995; Klein, 2002; Levine & Troiden, 1988). Referral to 12-step programs and therapy are made. Prematurely labeling a client as a sex addict can be damaging to the therapeutic relationship. Often, the discomfort of counselors to discuss sexual behaviors in a detailed manner results in premature labeling; thus, therapeutic opportunities for immediate intervention, treatment, and education are lost. I maintain that this approach to sexuality issues for the recovering substance abuser is simplistic in nature. A gross disservice is done with regard to addressing sexuality in a healthy manner and examining the development of beliefs and attitudes of individuals to assist in nonstigmatizing behavior change.

If treatment clinicians diagnose their clients as sexually addicted, they essentially lose an opportunity to treat them with clinically based interventions already in place. Some of these include medication and sex therapy based on individual physical and psychological assessment of clients as well as educational interventions (Schmidt, 1999). For clinicians to recommend that their clients take the alcohol and drug assessment but to substitute the words "sex" for "drugs and/or alcohol" and then refer them to 12-step recovery programs (such as Sex Addicts Anonymous) ignores the complexities of the issues involved and may cause psychological damage to individuals as well as additional stigma. Substance users already bear societal stigma based on their problematic chemical dependency, and adding another layer of stigma should not be done until more in-depth discussion of sexual behaviors is completed and assessed by sensitive and knowledgeable clinicians.

Caution in Interpreting Prevalence

The few studies that have examined out-of-control sexual behavior and substance abuse in young adults have revealed interesting results; one study (Seegers, 2003) found that 17.4 percent of men and 32.2 percent of women attending college met criteria indicating a need for sexual addiction treatment using the Sexual Addiction Screening Test (Carnes & O'Hara, 2000). These findings beg the question, How are so many young college students (women in particular) needing sexual addiction treatment?

To make a point, I took the Sexual Addiction Screening Test online at http://www.sexhelp.com/sast.cfm. The results revealed that I meet six criteria stating that sex addiction is present. I have a profile consistent with women who struggle with sexually compulsive behavior or a profile consistent with homosexual men who struggle with sexually compulsive behavior and also have the following dimensions of an addictive disorder appearing in my answers:

- Preoccupation: Obsessive thinking about sexual behavior, opportunities, and fantasies
- Relationship disturbance: Sexual behavior has created significant relationship problems
- Affect disturbance: Significant depression, despair, or anxiety over sexual behavior

This is interesting to consider, and I use this example to illustrate how its results can easily be misleading: I have been in a monogamous relationship for over eight years; I have no concerns with my sexual behavior but am curious how I would score; I am often preoccupied with sexual thoughts (as a sexologist working with sexual health, this is normal, but as a sexual being, I question why this would be considered abnormal); past relationships have led me to answer affirmatively for a few questions; of course I hide some of my sexual behaviors from others, as it is none of anyone's business what I do sexually in my relationship; I have felt degraded by my sexual behaviors (when I was forced to do things against my will in adolescence); I met my husband online, so I have used the Internet to make romantic or erotic connections with people online; I have subscribed to or regularly purchase or rent sexually explicit materials (I teach and conduct sex research and do this as part of my job); I regularly purchase romantic novel and sexually explicit magazines (for educational purposes); and I have stayed in romantic relationships after they became emotionally and physically abusive (being a survivor of domestic violence) to disclose a few pertinent scale item responses. The point I make here is that the questions on this instrument are very subjective and open to interpretation as well as moral judgment. Many of these behaviors are not necessarily indicative of problematic diagnoses but are behaviors that are condoned by conservative standards.

SEX ADDICTION LIMITATIONS

There is a lack of empirical data to support the neurological theories set forth in the field of sex addiction according to researchers Levine and

Troiden (1988) and Irvine (1995). They conclude that the field of sex addiction was socially constructed to fulfill the moral and financial goals of particular interest groups. Sex addiction theory evolved in the United States from the rise of culture and language of addiction (to chemicals), cultural tensions concerning sexuality (i.e., child molestation, pornography, or any perceived "deviant" sexual behaviors), and competing sexual ideologies within feminism (Irvine 1995). A large part of what deems behavior as unacceptable is dictated by social norms and acceptance. If a society or culture supports or rejects beliefs, this can set the stage for intolerance or rejection of certain behaviors, such as polyamorous relationships.

In relation to substance abuse, clusters of out-of-control sexual behaviors may occur together for people who demonstrate predispositions toward sexual sensation seeking or sexual compulsivity (Perera et al., 2009). For some people, sexually addictive behaviors occur only during episodes of substance use (Irons & Schneider, 1996). Some studies have shown that sensation seeking is associated with increased alcohol consumption and unprotected sex (Cyder, Flory, Rainer, & Smith, 2009; Norris et al., 2009). Differing relationships between use of specific substances and sexually compulsive behavior has been found to vary according to gender, but significant correlations do exist with regard to substance use and sexually compulsive behaviors (Eisenman, Dantzker, & Ellis, 2004).

There is a paucity of valid instruments to diagnose the concepts related to sexual sensation seeking and sexual compulsivity in general. Careful consideration of assessment in these areas is critical in substance abuse treatment. Improving sexual health in this population should include proper assessment, nonjudgmental attitudes and approaches of providers, and flexibility in the use of diagnostic criteria. If we use sensitivity and care in broaching the sexual behaviors of clients whose behaviors are at odds with the personal bias of providers, more appropriate interventions and referrals can be utilized. This will minimize further damage to our clientele.

SUGGESTED ACTIVITIES

A sexuality and addiction time line is a good activity for use in identifying and making connections to sexual abuse, rape, incest, problematic sexual behaviors, and substance use patterns. One way to facilitate such an activity is to spend one group session with clients in which they will explore their time line of substance abuse and sexual developmental milestones in a kinesthetic manner. Each client is given large butcher block paper, commonly called newsprint. Other materials include scissors, tape, glue sticks, marker, crayons, magazines, and assorted construction materials. They should be instructed to make their time line in any fashion deemed relevant to them. In other words, we don't want to impose a framework on them; they need to be able to create their own in ways that make sense to them.

I have utilized a similar activity in a life span development course with graduate students with great success for several years. The activity is conducted in two parts for the course. In one class meeting, they explore significant developmental milestones from birth through age 18, and in the second they repeat the process from age 18 to present. For use in a substance use setting, we would instruct clients to create the time line based from birth to present, noting areas such as age of onset for substance use, menstruation, puberty, first sexual experience, and any sexual experiences that were either positive or negative as well as a correlating time line of their substance use experiences.

The activity is best done in at least two 90-minute sessions. I would recommend allowing a full 40 to 45 minutes dedicated to the construction of the time line, leaving the last 45 minutes for some process of how it was for them to do this time line, what came up for them in terms of feelings, and what they noticed or remembered that they may have not realized in terms of connections to their substance use. I would also encourage clients to take home their time lines to work on in more depth over the next week so that if there were areas that were particularly painful or areas they may not have identified but were triggered in the discussion, they would have the opportunity to process the time line in their own space with more privacy. They should be informed that the following week, they will have the opportunity to share their timelines in group but are not required to do so—this allows for anonymity.

In the second session, facilitators also need to give clients permission to share or not share whatever they are comfortable with. It may not be appropriate for them to share deeply personal stories before they are ready. Again, meeting clients where they are at and not forcing them to share in a group until they feel prepared to do so is critical to the process of healing and not revictimizing them. The idea is gentle probing. Inevitably, some individuals will share a great deal; thus, the process piece can be very emotional and cathartic.

Time frames in individual presentation of the time lines should be observed, so depending on the size of the group (not more than 8 to 10 in a group is recommended at a time), 5 to 10 minutes would be the ideal time limit. Of course, observing this can be tricky, as we don't want to cut someone off if he or she is in a particularly vulnerable place. The facilitator needs to remind participants about the time limits of sharing both before starting and in between stories in order to help keep folks on track.

It is also recommended for comments and discussion to be held until the entire group has shared in order to keep moving through the activity. Depending on the length and intensity of sharing, this activity could be extended to three weeks, but two is optimal, as we want clients to be able to share the most pressing connections to their sexual selves and substance use, not their entire stories. Ask clients to limit their presentations to the most impactful connections between sexuality and substance abuse in order to focus them. Time lines should and could also be used for relapse prevention and treatment planning and may be used for individual sessions with the client's primary counselor if there are pressing issues that need more intensive exploration. In addition, journaling between sessions is another method for personal exploration.

TIME LINE CONNECTIONS

A shared sex and drug–linked connection that was discovered through facilitation of one of my sexuality groups illustrates the significance of using the sexuality time line. There were clear connections from sexual behavior and subsequent lying about it that resulted in feelings of shame. These discovered connections allowed this individual to further explore how the resulting shame from the sexual behavior was linked to her heroin use to cope:

Casey: I went down to Miami, my friend graduated from law school, and I met this guy and slept with him that night. I came back here to Chicago, maybe like a month later, and realized I was pregnant, but I had a boyfriend. So I told the boyfriend that I was pregnant, and just, like, pretended that it was his kid, and you know that really sucked. But it ended up being an ectopic pregnancy, so I didn't have the baby. But I was going to have the baby and tell this guy that it was his even though it wasn't his. It was shortly after all of that that we both started using heroin, and I never even thought about the connection before, but it's very close together.

Another client shared the following:

Linda: I was forced into having sex when I was 14; it wasn't my first time, but it was shortly thereafter. And because I didn't understand the definition of date rape, I didn't understand that's what it was for a few years, but I started using right around that time. I would say I actually started using and drinking before

that, so I think my body image had a lot to do with that because
I was very uncomfortable in my own skin; thus, drinking would
lower my inhibitions, and all of a sudden I felt prettier, I felt
skinnier, and I cared too much about who I was with or what
was going. The shame I felt from the rape I would say fueled the
need to numb the already negative feelings that were going on.

Feelings of shame are not necessarily caused by any specific situation
but rather by the person's interpretation of an event. The experience of
shame is a desire to hide, disappear, or die (Lewis, 1992). When shamed
repeatedly, people develop strategies to rid themselves of these feelings,
including depression, substance abuse, and/or acting-out behaviors.
Translated to our population, the results of being shamed from negative
sexual experiences needs to be addressed in order for clients to heal.

Through an examination of personal values and bias, we can begin to
objectively view the behaviors of clients with a broader perspective. Recognizing limitations of defining the more "controversial" sexuality topics
can assist providers in taking a less judgmental approach when communicating with clients and facilitating sexual health groups. Working with
more difficult topics, such as Internet sex, pornography use, and out-of-
control sexual behavior, is challenging but rewarding. Developing a positive approach will go a long way in fostering our relationships with clients
who are struggling with these issues.

RESOURCES

Books

Copeland, M. E., & Harris, M. (2000). *Healing the trauma of abuse: A
    women's workbook.* Oakland, CA: New Harbinger Publications.
Maltz, W. (2001). *The sexual healing journey.* New York: Harper.
Shapiro, F. (2004). *EMDR: The breakthrough therapy for overcoming
    anxiety, stress and trauma.* Cambridge, MA: Basic Books.

Online Resources

Institute for Sexual Wellness. http://www.instituteforsexualwellness.org.
National Council on Child Abuse and Family Violence. http://www
    .nccafv.org.
National Infertility Association: http://www.resolve.org.
Prevent Child Abuse America. http://www.preventchildabuse.org.
Rape, Abuse, and Incest National Network. http://www.rainn.org.

SEVEN

Body Beautiful

Inside yourself or outside, you never have to change what you see, only the way you see it.

—Thaddeus Golas

We are what we eat, isn't that what they say? We also live what we learn and learn what we are taught. If children are taught to despise their bodies and that their self-worth is tied to their looks, they will undoubtedly internalize feelings of self-loathing around body image. How many of us can look into the mirror and like what we see? If you are like me (or many people I know), you are always cutting yourself up into bits and pieces. This part needs work, that part needs toning, and if only I could rid myself of x number of pounds, then I would feel better about myself. Very few people are comfortable in their own bodies.

INFLUENCES ON BODY IMAGE

There are many influences in society that contribute to this body loathing. They include media, peer influence, and family. Media play a big role in perpetuating myths around beauty and attractiveness. All we have to do is turn on the television, open a magazine, or drive down the street, and we are bombarded with messages of what is desirable and what we need to do, fix, or buy in order to achieve that certain "look." Of course, messages about what is acceptable in culture changes over time. Early eighteenth- and nineteenth-century women were much larger and voluptuous than they are today, and this was the norm. Over time, this standard shifted, and with the coming of women's rights to vote and the women's movement for equality in the 1960s and 1970s, a backlash occurred. As women became larger through being able to have more power in society, they were expected to take up less physical space with their bodies. These images are portrayed through film and advertising, and although the changes may seem subtle and innocuous, the results are devastating. We see the results through the onset of eating disorders, compulsive exercise, and the use of products and pills to find ways to reduce our size and take up less space in the world.

Men are affected as well. Messages about what it means to be a man include adopting a macho stance, looking muscular and fit, and being aggressive to show a masculine guise. Having a large, muscular body is perceived as necessary to be able to back up the masculine image. The larger the body, the more menacing and able to garner respect the man is. In order to achieve this status, working out and taking muscle enhancers, steroids, or weight gainers is often perceived as needed. Any behavior that is obsessive or compulsive is potentially not healthy, especially if it leads to the use of addictive substances in order to achieve results.

DEFINITIONS

Body image is the perception someone has of his or her own body. Body image is an integral part of self-image and forms the basis of self-representation. Body image includes a set of images, fantasies, and meanings about the body, its parts, and its functions. It is affected by relationship with friends and family members, life experiences, and how they think others view them. The construct of body image has been defined as a multidimensional attitude toward one's body that includes perceptual, affective, and cognitive components. But the current emphasis of researchers on body image is on shape, weight, and the degree to which individuals are satisfied with their appearance (Cash, Ancis, & Strachan, 1997).

TYPES OF BODY IMAGE

There are several types of body image disturbances. These include anorexia (excessive caloric restriction), bulimia (eating large quantities of food, then purging [vomiting]), binge-eating disorder (consuming large quantities of food that cause excessive weight gain), and body dysmorphic disorder (where a person has minor or imaginary self-perceived physical flaws that cause him or her to compulsively obsess about one's appearance). Although there are differences in these disorders, they all share a common thread of general unhappiness with one's appearance. Some body image disturbances have more of a psychological cause, such as anorexia and body dysmorphic disorder, but all of them can result in negative health consequences.

BODY IMAGE ACROSS THE LIFE SPAN

Addressing negative body image is important because millions of people are affected on a daily basis and may engage in excessive, unhealthy behaviors in an effort to conform to the media's preconceived standard of body image. Because negative body image affects individuals across the life span, attention is needed to help those suffering learn that healthy bodies come in all shapes and sizes and that happiness does not come from adhering to societal expectations of the perfect body; rather, it comes from within. By helping individuals obtain and maintain a positive body image, the effects of depression, anxiety, low self-esteem, isolation, and even suicide can be minimized. A brief review of perceptions of body image over the life span is provided to assist the reader in conceptualizing developmental concerns. Selected client interviews are included in adult age ranges, including a group of individuals who were interviewed in each age range.

Children and Body Image (Ages 0 to 11)

While there is a wealth of information on children and body image, many statistics overlap. Some believe that basic body image is determined by age six. Media and peer groups tend to be prominent forces in influencing body image among young children. While the media, child care providers, teachers, and peers influence how children see themselves, the strongest determiner comes from how accepting parents/caregivers are of their own body. Adult role models, peers, and the mass media tend to be the common denominator when it comes to looking at the influences on how children view themselves.

Perceptions of one's body become increasingly important during adolescence as children experience multiple physical and social changes. Yet many children have a poor body image. Body dissatisfaction can develop by first grade, and girls tend to be less satisfied with their bodies compared to boys. Children as young as five years old have been treated for eating disorders. According to the National Eating Disorders

Association (2005), 42 percent of first through third graders said they wanted to be thinner. The U.S. Department of Health and Human Services (2009) cited that 80 percent of girls in grades 3 through 6 display body image concerns and dissatisfaction with appearance. Fifty percent of 9- and 10-year-olds feel better about themselves if they are on a diet. By fourth grade, 80 percent of American girls have dieted or are dieting. Eighty percent of 10-year-olds said they were afraid of being fat.

While these statistics concentrate more on girls than boys, new information is surfacing showing the struggles that preteen boys are facing as well. Between the world of sports and media portrayals of muscle and girth being the image of a "real" man, boys are becoming more concerned about achieving this look over intelligence, compassion, and emotional well-being (Natenshon, 2006). Knowing this, it becomes vital for parents and/or caregivers to recognize signs of a negative body image in their children. Along with being aware of signs and symptoms of depression, low self-esteem, or lack of involvement (indicators of an unhealthy body image), parents also need to listen to the language their children are using. Are their children describing themselves only in terms of their physical appearance? Do they talk about or show signs of excessive dieting? Do they make frequent comments about the weight of other children? If it becomes evident that a body image issue is visible, consulting the child's doctor is recommended (Natenshon, 2011).

Parental Influence

Parents and caregivers can make a difference in encouraging a positive body image in their children by being aware of their attitudes about body shape and weight. It is important for parents to stay away from making negative comments about their or others' bodies, and to avoid stereotypes and prejudices associated with weight. Parents can help their children understand that their bodies will grow and change and that there is not one "ideal" body shape. Talking about being healthy and what our bodies help us do, along with discussing the unrealistic media images and concentrating on role models, are ways to shift the focus from physical appearance to inner strengths (Kearney-Cooke, 2002).

Adolescents to Young Adults (Ages 12 to 24)

Anxiety about weight and unhealthy lifestyle habits diminish the self-esteem and integrity of growing children while consuming attention and energy that is needed for other important developmental tasks. A compelling wish to be slim provides the seeds for many body image, eating, fitness, and weight problems that are extremely difficult to reverse once established, including a rising rate of fatness. While much remains to be learned, enough is now known about the toxic messages that promote body image and weight concerns to prevent these problems before they start.

Too many young individuals ages 12 to 24 suffer from unhealthy body image. A large percentage of adolescent girls (50 to 88%) feel negatively about their bodies, while 58 percent of girls want to lose weight (Croll, 2007). Family, friends, media, or other outside sources can and may contribute greatly to the way that adolescents view themselves physically. Even at such a young age, individuals pay too much attention to how their bodies may appear different than their peers: whether their waist is wider or rounder, their thighs look thicker, they are shorter or taller, and their butt is a little smaller or flatter than their best friends. Having an extreme focus on one's body image can lead to major physical, emotional, social, and psychological concerns. These concerns could include extreme diets, use and abuse of weight loss pills or diuretics, excessive weight loss or weight gain, loss of social network, anorexia, bulimia, depression, and so on. Roughly 70 percent of adolescent girls eat in unhealthy, restrictive ways for the purpose of controlling or losing weight (U.S. Department of Health and Human Services, 2009). This is extending to younger and younger children. Furthermore, 66 percent of adolescent girls and 21 percent of adolescent boys are compromising their nutritional needs out of fear of becoming fat (Croll, 2007). At such a young age, children are preventing proper body growth because of potential diets or food restrictions. By providing interventions for those suffering as well as educating family members or loved ones, we could help to prevent such issues from arising and educate outsiders affected by the severity of such a widespread issue.

Parental Influence

Parents and the media can be very influential when dealing with children, adolescents, and young adults. Magazines, television, and other forms of media revealed that women's magazine ads promoted 10.5 times more weight loss than men's (National Association of Social Workers, 2001). It is important for parents to help promote a healthy body image in their teens. Although our teens are being bombarded with messages about how "imperfect" their bodies are, there are still many things parents can do to promote a positive body image. Helping to educate adults or caregivers on the proper way to help reduce or eliminate low body image can be the first step to prevention (U.S. Department of Health and Human Services, 2009).

One can follow these steps to help adolescents and young adults or loved ones to develop a positive body image and relate to food in a healthy way (Poncelet, 2009): (1) make sure your child understands that weight gain is a normal part of development, especially during puberty; (2) avoid negative statements about food, weight, and body size and shape; (3) allow your child, adolescent, or young adult to make decisions about food while making sure that plenty of healthy and nutritious meals and snacks are available; (4) compliment your child or adolescent on his or her efforts, talents, accomplishments, and personal values; (5) restrict television viewing and watch television with your child or adolescent and discuss the media images you see; (6) encourage your school to enact policies against size and sexual discrimination, harassment, teasing, and name-calling and support the elimination of public weigh-ins and fat measurements; and (7) keep the communication lines with your child open so the or she knows that you are always there for him or her (U.S. Department of Health and Human Services, 2009).

Early and Middle Adults (Ages 25 to 59)

Although much research exists on body image in children, adolescents, and college students, few studies have examined body image dissatisfaction in adults. Research needs to be expanded to adults to determine what influences body satisfaction and dissatisfaction have in adulthood. Studies show that even in early and middle adulthood, personal appearance is important and influences how we feel about ourselves and how we interact with others. The media continue to influence how we view beauty even as we get older. Because the media stress being thin, most children and adults equate attractiveness to thinness. Women strive for the thin, toned body, while men strive for the strong, muscular body. Approximately 7 million females and 1 million males struggle with eating disorders, 25 percent of males and 45 percent of females are on a diet on any given day, Americans spend over $40 billion on dieting and diet-related products each year, and 80 percent of woman are dissatisfied with their appearance (National Eating Disorders Association, 2005).

Body image continues to be influenced by family, friends and romantic partners, culture, size prejudice, health professionals, and the media. Adults who come from families where the parents obsessed about their body weight or imposed food restrictions were more like to develop a poor body image. Similarly, weight- or shape-related criticism by family members or others has been found to contribute significantly to body dissatisfaction. At work or in group living situations, adults may be surrounded by negative body talk. Constantly hearing negative comments about your-self or others can create a feeling of self-conscious about one's body, even if the adult was not worried about it in the past. Males and females may feel pressured to be thin or muscular in order to be accepted by a potential romantic partner.

Client Experiences

One of my sexuality group members in this age range stated,

Um, I think a big part of why I used was due to body image, um. I've never been comfortable with my own image of what I've had of myself, and that's a lot of what played a part of my family and the guys that I dated. Constantly, the men in my life told me that you need to lose weight, you need to dress like this, you need to act like that, so that really lowered my self-esteem, and I already had a low self-esteem as it was. So I used the drugs as a way to cope with those emotional pains that I had but also to reach my goal of the body weight; that was a big reason for a lot of my [drug] relapses because I've gained the weight back and that I was told those things again. So I would use because it would instantly make me lose, like, all the weight.

Cultural Influences

Culture influences adults, as American society places an emphasis on weight, size, and appearance. Similarly, men and women are exposed to size prejudice where thin and muscular is equated with being hard-working, successful, popular, beautiful, strong, and self-disciplined and being fat or heavyset is equated with being lazy, ignorant, hated, ugly, weak, and lacking willpower. Routine doctor visits can cause a change in body image as height and weight measurements are taken and assigned a certain label: underweight, average weight, overweight and obese. Health professionals may even encourage an adult to lose weight based on what the "ideal" height and weight charts says the individual should weigh, and not take into consideration other factors, such as muscle mass (which weighs more than fat), large bone structure and genetics.

Media Influences

Even though the media portray unrealistic body images, men and women strive to achieve what they have been conditioned to accept as normal or acceptable body size, weight, and shape. But only 5 percent of the women have the genetic makeup to achieve and maintain this image. The media depict males to have bulging muscles and females to be thin and attractive. In real life, GI Joe would be 5 feet 10 inches and have a 55-inch chest and a 27-inch bicep (this is larger than most professional competitive bodybuilders), and Barbie would be 5 feet 9 inches and weigh 110 pounds with measurements of 39/18/33 and would be unable to menstruate because of low body fat. Over the last 25 years, what is considered "normal" has gotten thinner for woman and more muscular for men. The average model use to weigh 8 percent less than the average American woman but today weighs 23 percent less. A *Playgirl* centerfold model of 1976 would need to shed 12 pounds of fat and gain 27 pounds of muscle to be a centerfold today (Leit, Pope, & Gray, 2001).

Client Experiences

Negative influences and unrealistic expectations have played a role in both males and females having a distorted self-image. Males see themselves as thinner and less muscular than they really are. The drive for muscularity in young men has been associated with self-esteem, neuroticism, and perfectionism. It may also influence men to use or abuse anabolic steroids to achieve their goals. One study found that females overestimate the size of their hips by 16 percent and their waists by 25 percent, yet these same women were able to correctly estimate the width of a box. The perception that they are bigger than they really are can often lead to eating disorders, obsessive exercising, and drug use (Wilcox, 1997). Consider this case:

I think for body image, well, throughout life I always like wanted to be thinner than what I was, and for me, using cocaine and meth was the perfect solution to that problem, and I'm 5 feet 10 inches, and I was all the way down to 119 and I've been all the way up to 210, and my weight just, in the last five years just like totally fluctuates like completely like way up and way down very quickly, so for me, like yea. I've identified that weight is going to be my big thing that I'm going to have to watch when I leave here that might cause me to go back to it and all the other stuff, like, I'm not comfortable with where I'm at now, which is a completely comfortable weight especially for my height, but I'm just kind of weird about that. But I also think that I also used alcohol and other drugs to just be comfortable in sexual situations because I'm never comfortable; even when I'm looking the way I want to, I'm not comfortable. I'm not comfortable with sex, and I think my body image got better for me when I got some tattoos and piercing and felt that that made my body more like mine and I felt more comfortable in my own skin, but I've never been comfortable in sexual situations with regard to my body.

Adult Statistics

Statistics for early and middle adults show that two out of five women and one out of five men would trade three to five years of their life to achieve their weight goals. This can lead to extreme behaviors with regard to weight management. Thirty-five percent of occasional dieters progress into pathological dieting. The bulk of male body issues appear between the ages of 45 and 55, with men showing insecurities about their stomachs, chests, and hair loss (Rand & Wright, 2000).

Findings based on interviews conducted with adults ages 25 to 59 indicated that there were many similarities and a few differences in body image for males and females. Similarities in men and woman indicated that favorite body parts made up features that would not change with weight (i.e., lips, eyes, dimples, and hands), that the least favorite body part was indicative of something they wanted to change because of size or scarring, and that no one in the interviews would consider surgery or Botox to change their bodies was striking. Both men and women indicated that their personal body image was influenced by family and/or media and that their view of themselves would change if they lost a limb or breast/testicle. But if their partner lost a limb or breast/testicle, their view of their partner would *not* change. When asked about how they were different from or similar to theirs, everyone named personality traits rather than body parts. The one difference that the interviews established between males and females were that men wanted to gain weight and be more muscular and that women wanted to lose weight or return to their prechildbearing weight.

The Older Generation (Ages 60 to Infinity)

As of 2011, 78 million members of the baby boom generation, those folks born from 1946 through 1964, will be turning 65. That means that the population of American adults in this age-group will almost double between 2005 and 2030 to more than 70 million, almost 20 percent of the population (National Institute on Aging, 2006). Most often, issues that come to mind for this older group are health care, financial security, depression, grief, family dynamics, and so on. Very little attention seems to be paid to the apprehension or distress of the "body image." This section addresses the myriad concerns that face the older generation, those 60 and older, in both a scientific and a personal manner. Specific mention is made detailing the range of body worries/satisfaction, body discomforts, anxiety about the aging body, health practices to obtain/maintain the body, and cognitive control and gender observations.

The prevalence of body dissatisfaction is being termed a "normative discontent." What this suggests is that it is an extremely common trait at any age to be anxious about the body to some degree. Negative body image and body dissatisfaction have been implicated as risk factors for various forms of psychopathology, including depression, anxiety, and disordered eating (Forman & Davis, 2005). What these participants have determined as they uncovered many aspects of each age-group is that it is universal. In other words, the greatest stressor may still be among the older faction, but it is merging ever more into the younger generations (even to the very young). Most of the people interviewed in the older group stated that they are concerned about how their bodies are regressing at an unequal pace as their minds or attitudes. They were not negatively influenced by the media or what some would consider superficial influences. They were more persuaded by family and friends (and even their doctors).

Aging, Biology, and Body Image

Biological changes in the body play a role in how healthy lifestyles are practiced among the aging population. Menopause is associated with a number of body-related changes, including increased weight and a slowed metabolism, that contrast with ideals of physical appearance and may contribute to body dissatisfaction. The literature on clinical eating disorders that were diagnosed for the first time after menopause is limited. Late-onset eating disorder symptoms might be a response to biological changes associated with aging. Perhaps one of the more prominent culture-based risk factors for older women is the fear of aging. It is reasonable that women experience greater concern over aging than men because it represents a percieved loss of attractiveness.

Aging, Gender, and Body Image

Despite the noted lack of empirical research on body image and eating disorders in older adults, there appears to be an emerging consensus on some aspects. Women experience high levels of body dissatisfaction, that this dissatisfaction persists across the life span, and that women continually report more dissatisfaction with their body than do men. While body dissatisfaction appears stable, the importance placed on physical appearance tends to decrease over time (Peat, Peyerl, & Muehlenkamp, 2008).

Women tend to have a significantly increased level of dissatisfaction, anxiety, and discomfort about their aging. It should also be noted that women appear to engage in or promote more of a positive healthy lifestyle as they age. Instead of comparing themselves to individuals in their social networks, older persons might compare their current state with that of when they were younger (Peat et al., 2008). Another observation suggests that older women do suffer from eating disorders that warrant intervention, yet their eating disorders may be misdiagnosed or left untreated.

To no great surprise, there exists an overall lack of research on men, particularly older men. Men of all ages tend to experience less anxiety and displeasure than women with regard to body image. Evidence is emerging that proposes that as age increases, there is greater tolerance in what body sizes are considered acceptable. It appears that although older adults may be more accepting of a range of body types in others, they still might perceive their own body type as unacceptable and may experience body dissatisfaction. Having this awareness of older adults in treatment may assist counselors in identifying body image issues when present.

CONNECTIONS TO SUBSTANCE MISUSE

Body image development is an important element of the developmental process, and skewed messages can contribute to substance use and misuse. Poor body image has been identified as a risk factor for substance abuse. Poor body image among adolescents is associated with greater substance use. For adolescents with poor body image due to weight, substance use may be a weight control strategy (Nieri, Kulis, Keith, & Hurdle, 2005).

Substance Use as Coping Strategy

Substance use also may be a coping strategy for adolescents whose severe body image problems are manifest in eating disorders. Numerous studies have documented the co-occurrence of eating disorders and substance abuse. Typically, the eating disorder is accompanied by poor body image and precedes the substance use, and the presence of the former tends to accelerate the development of the latter. Wilson (1999) argued that eating disorders do not indicate an addiction to food or represent a larger problem of addictive behavior. Rather, substance use may be a coping strategy for dealing with the negative effects of eating disorders. For instance, binge eaters may use substances to alleviate their emotional distress and the physical discomfort associated with starvation between binges.

Substance use also has been found to accompany early stage eating disorder symptoms, such as frequent dieting, that often coincide with low body esteem. For example, an association between cigarette and alcohol use and disordered eating for boys and girls and an association between binge drinking and disordered eating for boys was found (Croll, Neumark-Sztainer, Story, & Ireland, 2002). Dieting in the sixth grade predicted alcohol use in the ninth grade in middle school boys and girls living in Wisconsin (Krahn et al., 1996). In a study of over 33,000 adolescent boys and girls living in Minnesota, weekly or daily alcohol or tobacco use was about one and a half times more prevalent in youth who always dieted compared with youth who never dieted (French, Perry, Leon, & Fulkerson, 1994). The most frequent dieters had the poorest body image, whereas the youth who never dieted had the most positive body image.

The presence of substance use among individuals with early stage eating disorder symptoms was also documented (Granner & Black, 2001). In their sample of African American and Caucasian college women, individuals with high levels of body dissatisfaction and a strong drive for thinness were more likely to report cigarette use and binge drinking. No racial differences were found in the relationship between eating disorder symptoms and substance use.

The findings from studies using subclinical samples suggest that substance use among adolescents with poor body image may be a more general coping strategy. This concept is supported by the findings of other studies linking poor body image to low self-esteem and depression, each of which are risk factors for substance use (Kinnier, Metha, Okey, & Keim, 1994; Scheier, Botvin, Griffin, & Diaz, 2000; Siegel, 2002). Adolescents with poor body image may turn to substance use as an escape from their feelings of low self-worth and depression.

Social Acceptance

Substance use also may be a perceived avenue toward social acceptance. Youth who dislike their looks or body and assume that their peers feel the same about them may believe that using substances will make them more attractive socially. This argument was made to explain findings of substance-using, dieting adolescents (French et al., 1994). The researchers suggested that these adolescents engage in risk behaviors to establish social contacts and win approval from peers. Based on the developmental recommendations earlier in this chapter, the sooner parents can foster healthy body image, the less susceptible to substance abuse their children and adolescents may be.

Gender, Body Image, and Substance Misuse

Disliking one's looks appears to be more of a risk factor for boys than for girls. Boys may turn to substance use to compensate for their perceived unattractiveness. Certainly, the pervasive media images, such as in the alcohol advertising geared toward males, associate substance use with a variety of positive traits, including male attractiveness, especially toward the other gender. Some boys may believe or hope that substance use can enhance their image. Alternatively, these boys may simply use substances to ease their discomfort with their appearance during social interactions (French et al., 1994).

For girls, on the other hand, weight-related body image appears to be a more salient predictor of substance use (Croll et al., 2002). Not surprisingly, the substance associated with body image for girls is cigarettes, which are commonly believed to control weight. This finding supports the notion that some girls may use substances as a weight control strategy (Boles & Johnson, 2001). Although boys who viewed themselves as too thin reported greater lifetime cigarette use and weaker antidrug norms, their concerns may be less about weight than about size or build. By smoking, these boys may believe that they project a tough, masculine image, sufficient to compensate for what they perceive to be lacking physically in stature or musculature. These results are consistent with previous research suggesting that weight-related concerns are more common among girls and that size/build concerns are more common among boys (Raudenbush & Zellner, 1997).

Substance Misuse and Weight Attainment

For some people, in order to achieve their desired body, drugs will be misused. Steroid use to attain muscle mass is more prevalent in men than women. Weight loss strategies, such as restricting food and caloric intake, can be enhanced through amphetamine use. Developing other disordered patterns of weight loss are other risks associated with addiction, such as the use of diuretics, compulsive exercise, or bingeing and purging.

For those who suffer from binge-eating disorders and obesity, there can be some adaptive advantages of engaging in these behaviors and maintaining a high weight. Associations between child sexual abuse and obesity have been documented in research studies. In these cases, some victims gain weight as a protective factor—they intuitively know that excessive weight gain will reduce the number of sexual advances from potential partners, and this may be appealing for some. For other individuals, losing weight can be a potential relapse trigger, as reaching a weight at which they were abused may trigger posttraumatic stress disorder symptoms and subsequent drug use. It is important to be aware of past abuse histories of overweight clients in order to bring this awareness to them and help develop a comprehensive relapse prevention plan. Some clients have difficulties in losing weight past a certain point because of this unconscious mental barrier associated with past abuse.

Client Experiences

Interviews with several clients revealed differing weight associations. One person's first attempt at recovery was sabotaged by links to weight gain and loss. The client had previously been a competitive bodybuilder and used amphetamines and exercise to achieve his ideal weight and look. After leaving treatment, this client relapsed when preparing to compete in a bodybuilding show. The association with weight loss was directly connected to the substance use. In order to recover, this person had to make the choice to lead another lifestyle, one that did not include competitive bodybuilding or dieting. A couple of years into recovery, the client stated, "No matter how good I looked on the outside, I still felt like killing myself."

Another example is of a client who had gained weight beyond where she was comfortable. Attempts at losing weight were futile, and weight loss below a certain number could not be achieved without relapse. On further examination, it was discovered that recent abuse at the lower weight was associated with the subsequent relapses. Dealing with the past abuse was recommended before any further weight loss attempts. Helping clients feel okay about their self-image, regardless of what their weight is, is a critical piece of the recovery process. A nice way to conceptualize this was stated by yet another client: "You can't make the insides feel good by making the outsides look good. That is an inside job . . . once my self-esteem improved, I was able to develop healthier eating and exercise patterns."

Body Image and Partner Attraction

As noted early on, the circles of Sexual Beingness are connected as well. In terms of body image issues, there are direct links to relationships, intimacy, and sexualization. As sexualization has to do with the use of one's sexuality to influence or manipulate others, flirting is a seemingly harmless concept that falls under sexualization. Flirting is a tool that people use to send out signals to others to let them know that they are attracted to them. For individuals who have low self-esteem, particularly young women, finding meaning through relationships with others is a source of comfort and security. And one way to attract potential mates is through the display of one's body; the more attractive and seductive one can be to potential partners, the more likely one is to be successful in obtaining one's choice of a mate.

Using one's body to get emotional, physical, and financial needs met is not a new practice. But when people go to any length to attract a partner, unhealthy behavioral patterns may emerge, including those that may put their health at risk. One client shared, "I knew from an early age that I could get anything I wanted by being sexual with men. If I gave them what they wanted, I got things in return." This particular individual did not prostitute herself in the stereotypical manner, but trading sex for favors or attention can have equally devastating results. After years of exchanging one's "personal" wares for security and relationships, a person internalizes their perceptions of self-worth. And if that self-worth is directly attached to how one looks, any other personal attributes the individual may have had in the past become useless. And if the pursuit of obtaining wealth and status become attached to practices associated with bartering the body for trade, a sense of personal value is diminished. We see the practice in young trophy wives who marry older men in exchange for status and power. In other cases, marriage itself can be the trade-off when individuals marry for money, not personal happiness and well-being. And when people are not happy because they have devalued themselves, a sense of shame can emerge that can be a big trigger for substance misuse.

Addressing Body Image in Treatment

Developing curricula and specific lessons for body image issues can aid counselors in fostering more positive body esteem in their clients. Again, once connections are identified between body esteem and substance abuse, lessons can be tailored to fit the group's particular needs. Reducing negative feelings of body loathing and finding ways for clients to embrace themselves—all of themselves—for who they are will go a long way in facilitating a healthier recovery process. The following activity can serve as a starting point for body attitude exploration and provide an understanding of the gender messages attached to them.

SAMPLE LESSON

Goal: Participants will learn how their self-image affects sexual decision making. Participants will learn how communication about sexual thoughts, needs, and feelings affect relationship dynamics.

Lesson Rationale: In American society, we are bombarded with media images of sexual perfection. These images are portrayed in a distorted manner, such as to be attractive, one must be thin, voluptuous, and beautiful (for women) and muscular, rugged looking, and handsome (for men). The internalization of how one should look with regard to body size can cause much shame, self-hatred, low self-esteem, and poor sexual boundary setting as a result. This inability to communicate about sexual thoughts, needs, and feelings can contribute to poor sexual decision making and high-risk sexual behavior. By looking at these issues in a non-threatening atmosphere, individuals can begin to redefine their attitudes toward what is healthy for them in relationships based on their own feelings and ideas, not those portrayed in a one-sided manner.

Time: 90 minutes

Objectives: Participants will do the following:

- Identify one area of body image that causes pain, shame, and/or confusion
- Identify one area of body image that causes joy, pleasure, or satisfaction
- Examine how internalized messages regarding body image can be used to influence and/or manipulate others
- Develop awareness of how one's actions may send messages that one may not intend to send

Materials:

- Prepared newsprint with the following headings; "sexy/attractive" (women), "sexy/attractive" (men), "not sexy/unattractive" (women), "not sexy/unattractive" (men)
- Markers
- Blank newsprint sheets (enough for one for each group)
- Circles of sexuality sheets
- Sentence completions
- Box of art supplies: ribbons, magazines, construction paper, stickers, glitter, markers, pens, and so on

Journal Share (20 minutes):
Facilitate journal sharing among group members from the previous week's sentence completions (this is a typical way to begin groups already in process).

Body Image Exercise (45 minutes):

1. Introduce the lesson by explaining that our self-image plays a big part in sexual decision making, how we choose out partners and why, whether we decide to be sexual, and how we take care of ourselves (or not) with regard to our bodies. Let them know in the next exercise that they are going to examine how they feel about themselves and others in terms of what makes someone appealing or not, identify areas they like and dislike about their own bodies, and think about ways they can change their thinking with regard to body image.

2. Distribute the four prepared sheets to four groups of participants. If there are only six people, divide the group in half and give each group two sheets. Optimally, there should be two to four participants per sheet, depending on the size of the group. Instruct them to list attributes that they feel make men and women sexy/attractive or not sexy/unattractive. Give them about 15 minutes to complete the lists. Encourage discussion among the groups and help them think about what is attractive (or not) to them as individuals, not just a group consensus.

3. When the groups are done, have the sexy/attractive sheets report first, reading their lists to the large group. Ask if anyone wishes to add to the lists. Use the following questions for process:
   a. Why did you choose these attributes?
   b. What about these attributes makes them appealing (or not)?
   c. How might this list look different in another culture or part of the world?
   d. What or who defines beauty in society?
   e. How are our perceptions of beauty connected to substance use?

4. Next, have the groups with not sexy/unattractive read their lists. Ask if anyone would like to add anything. Use the following questions for process:
   a. Why did you choose these attributes?
   b. How could this list be harmful to individuals?
   c. Could any of these attributes be viewed as sexy/attractive? Why or why not?
   d. Where do our beliefs around what is attractive come from?

e. How might substance use affect how we behave with regard to a negative body image?

5. Ask the group how they think men might have answered differently, if at all, than they did (or vice versa if this is a group of men). How do what men think about attractiveness influence women's feelings around what they view as attractive? Quickly brainstorm how might this play out in how they decide to behave sexually if they are the following:

   a. Beautiful/handsome
   b. Feel they are ugly or fat
   c. Lonely
   d. Want to be sexual with someone (horny)
   e. Stoned on drugs or drunk

6. Try to get them to identify behaviors of seduction or manipulation that women or men might engage in to influence others. Give examples if necessary to stimulate the brainstorm (i.e., flirting, dressing seductively, feeling powerful, having sex when they don't really want to, and so on). Facilitator should write their responses on a sheet of newsprint.

Evaluation/Homework (10 minutes):
Ask participants to fill out circles of sexuality sheet and answer the following questions on the back:

• What is one thing about your body that you don't like and why?
• What is one thing you like about your body and why?
• What are your personal triggers and connections with body image and substance use?

Hand out journal ideas (should coincide with lesson) for homework and go over instructions for the next assignment (not listed here) and provide ideas for creativity, such as drawings, collage, poems, and so on. Have the box of supplies ready and let group members pick items from it to use for their projects. Group members will be asked to start thinking of positive ideas connected to body image and to bring those ideas to group for the following lesson (five minutes).

PARTING THOUGHTS

Sobriety is about living life fully and completely, and sexual recovery is integral to the fullness of life. The first step toward change is awareness.

In their addiction, many people are not aware how much their sexual beings have been harmed by society's messages about what it means to be a male or female. Often, issues of body image, sexualization, and identity can lead to relapse. Becoming aware of body image and connections to substance use early in recovery can assist individuals in preventing relapse later on.

RESOURCES

Books

Atkins, Dawn, (Ed.). (1998). *Looking queer: Body image and identity in lesbian, bisexual, gay, and transgender communities.* New York: Haworth Press.

Cash, T. F., & Pruzinsky, T. (2002). *Body image: A handbook of theory, research and clinical practice.* New York: Guilford Press.

Online Resources

National Eating Disorders Association. http://www.nationaleating disorders.org.

Our Bodies Ourselves Health Resource Center. http://www.ourbodies ourselves.org/book/chapter.asp?id=1.

EIGHT

Self-Love and Dreams

In the nineteenth century masturbation was a disease; in the twentieth, it is a cure.

—Unknown

Graze on my lips; and if those hills be dry, stray lower, where the pleasant fountains lie.

—William Shakespeare

Whacking off, spanking the monkey, choking the chicken, polishing the pearl, paddling the pink canoe, rubbin' the nubbin, muffin buffin', priming the pump, rosy palm and her five sisters—whatever you call it, there are a lot of ways to refer to masturbation without actually saying the word.

As we move well into the twenty-first century, masturbation, although shown to be a healthy form of sexual expression, still remains stigmatized. In the 1950s, Alfred Kinsey and his research team shocked the world after showing how common and nonpathological the taboo sexual behavior was. Since then, masturbation has successfully been recognized as a legitimate means for improving sexual satisfaction and treating sexual dysfunctions. The inclusion of recreational sex as a form of self-pleasure is also discussed here in the framework of treatment.

ORIGINS OF HISTORICAL VIEWS

Early civilizations had differing views on the act of masturbating, ranging from positive to sinful. Sex was necessary for procreation. Any other aspects of sexual behavior that detracted from procreation were condemned and prohibited in many religious systems. St. Augustine, the major formulator of Western Christian attitudes on sexual issues, actually suffered from sexual compulsion based on his autobiography where he prayed to God to save him from his sexual sins—but not yet! It has been common for religious zealots to vehemently condemn behaviors with which they personally struggle. With St. Augustine's conversion to Christianity, he deemed that the only acceptable sexual behaviors were of a procreative nature; any other kind of sexual activity was forbidden and sinful, as was use of any barriers to contraception. Augustine actually advocated for tolerance of prostitution over masturbation for those men who could not find or support a suitable wife. Without prostitution, the men would turn to homosexuality, masturbation, and other, more sinful activities (Bullough, 1976).

Following the development of Protestantism, the Catholic Church continued to give prominence to the evils of masturbation, emphasizing its relationship to sodomy, deserving of severe penalties. "Sex, outside of the missionary position in marital intercourse, was somehow impure, and if pleasure resulted from it, it was highly immoral and was to be avoided" (Bullough, 2001, p. 27). Deep controversies arose between Catholicism and Protestantism, with the latter forming a critical stance over the treatment of "sexual offenses" in marriage. As the power of religious authorities began to wane with regard to these divides (mainly nonprocreative sexual behaviors), the developments of medicine and the medical model in the seventeenth and eighteenth centuries continued to fuel fears and confirmed the dangers of masturbation with "scientific data." Medical theories were competing to explain certain diseases that were attributed to these perceived sexual "deviant" behaviors prior to discoveries regarding germs and bacteriology.

The effects of the loss of semen on the body were the focus of several famous European physicians, and then others joined in, resulting in the labeling of all nonprocreative sexual activity as onanism (derived from a biblical story about Onan's sin of wasting his seed for not wanting to marry his dead brother's wife). Masturbation was blamed for consequences of sexually transmitted diseases, as well as any form of nonprocreative sex, and resulted in an age that was dubbed "masturbatory insanity." This continued into the nineteenth century with an onslaught of literature warning from the "authorities" about the dangers of masturbation as well as popular books for parents to help them recognize signs of masturbation in their children and teenagers (of course, all warning behaviors were, in fact, normal child and adolescent behaviors). The panic resulted in the invention of literally dozens of mechanical antimasturbatory devices and procedures, including cutting foreskin of the penis to cause pain if rubbed, a hot iron to a girl's clitoris to scar it and prevent masturbation, burning topical ointments, binding children's hands at night under bedding, clitoridectomies (cutting off the clitoris), cutting of the labia, and male castration, to name a few (although few physicians resorted to the most drastic of the measures). One of the most lasting "cures" for boys was circumcision so that the foreskin did not have to be pulled back for cleaning and tempt him to masturbate.

Changes slowly began to come about with the development of a germ theory and the discovery of the agents that actually caused gonorrhea and syphilis. Further research on the prevalence of masturbation across race, gender, and culture also challenged some of the myths, as did the increased investigation of sex research. Consequences of masturbation were more dependent on a mind-set than on any tangible data. The sexual revolution in the 1960s gave way to new sources of information and reassessment of sexual attitudes and values in the United States. Masturbation was not only approved but also recommended to be used as an important technique in sex therapy (Kaplan, 1975). Views shifted from masturbation as a dangerous sin to a "virtue by which individuals could promote their well-being and skills for sexual interaction" (Kontula & Haavio-Mannila, 2002, p. 53). Despite the positive shifts in perspective, much stigma associated with masturbation still remains as we consider the firing of an American surgeon general for speaking positively about masturbation in the Clinton administration. There is clearly more work to be done.

THREE COMPETING VIEWS OF SEXUAL BEHAVIORS

Three normative but competing views of sexual behaviors currently exist in the United States and can be attributed, in part, to the origins and conflicts that resulted from more modern and less erroneous views of masturbation. These views are procreative, relational, and recreational.

Procreational

Religious doctrine guides the procreative view. Within the procreative (heterosexual) view is the concept of monogamy, that is, one man/one woman and no others. Historically, upper-class citizens were allowed to have nonmonogamous relationships; monogamy was forced on lower-class citizens and slaves in order to control their relationships. So, in effect, religious sanctions enforced control over people through this perspective through the institution of marriage. Interestingly enough, over 15 different sexual lifestyles have been identified as existing within societies (Stayton, 1985). Traditional monogamous relationships do not constitute the majority of these either, but with sparse data on prevalence, accurate estimates are difficult to assess.

Relational

Strict adherence to legally or religiously sanctioned relationships does not guide the relational view of sexual pleasure. Masturbation can occur in marriage or relationships either solo or mutually shared. As a dimension of a stable or growing relationship, sexual expression has been termed "relational." Relational sexual expression has been described as a manifestation of a multifaceted relationship of sharing and communicating. Intimacy is more than physical; it has meaning intrinsic to the experience and is a full sharing of oneself with another (Kelly & Freysinger, 2000).

Recreational

Recreational views of sex are more liberal and not confined to a stable or committed relationship. Recreational sex is just that: sex for pleasure. When we examine human behavior in general, it can be driven by social norms and/or biological urges. Within these two camps is much dissension. If we ask the question, What is the purpose of human sexuality, for reproduction or pleasure? the answer includes both and more. From a physiological viewpoint, it has been postulated that reproduction may just be a by-product of sexual pleasure. Sex as leisure or recreation suggests that sex is primarily for the experience itself and not necessarily connected with some deeper meaning. And with regard to monogamy, it does not exist in any species naturally. Some pairing exists within animal and bird species, but sex with other animals and birds (non-monogamous sexual behaviors) within the species occurs. Humans are the only species that had to go get all hung up about trying to control one another's sexual behavior.

Forms of Relational and Recreational Sex

Within the recreational (and relational) views of sex, sexual pleasure can take many forms, including partnered sexual behaviors (sexual intercourse, oral sex, and manual stimulation of genitals), other sexual behaviors (watching erotic videos, playing erotic games, viewing online pornography, going to strip clubs, masturbation, reading erotic material, anal intercourse, and participating in threesomes), as well as recreational/hedonistic sexual behaviors (living for the moment when it comes to sex, having sex for fun, enjoying new exciting sexual experiences/sensations, enjoying wild uninhibited sexual encounters, viewing sex as a recreational activity, and experimenting with new sexual behaviors). We cannot always separate relational and recreational sex, as many of these so-called recreational behaviors can and do take place within committed and stable relationships. How can this be? you might be asking. This brings us to a related facet of sexual health directly related to masturbation and recreational sex: fantasy.

THE STUFF THAT DREAMS ARE MADE OF

Everyone dreams and fantasizes from time to time, from wishful thinking to winning the lottery and escape to other realities. Some of the most common fantasies are about romantic and sexual encounters, and in fact sexual fantasies are normal and encouraged in U.S. culture.

Take, for example, the fairy tale of Cinderella or other childhood stories whose hopeful endings are "happily ever after." These are the blueprints for what women are socialized to dream about. Or take beer commercials where all the women are beautiful and hanging all over the man as he drinks to his heart's content. Have one of these (beer), and you will attract multiple beautiful women who will fawn over your sexual prowess.

The Role of Sexual Fantasy

Understanding sexual fantasies seem central to understanding an important part of human sexuality for a couple of reasons. In addition to the fact that they are nearly universally experienced, they can affect later sexual behavior as well as reflect past experience. As with the chicken-and-egg syndrome, a person's fantasies can be affected by what they have read or seen as well as be influenced to act on sexual fantasies through behaviors. In fantasy, one is free to imagine whatever they wish, however unrealistic, without experiencing embarrassment, rejection, or societal or legal restrictions; thus, they can be completely harmless and healthy and provide avenues for sexual exploration and enjoyment of sexual pleasure.

So, an individual might fantasize about same sex exploration or sex with more than one person and then take action to engage in the experience. The level of social acceptance of the behaviors coupled with internalized messages regarding the behavior will affect how well this person might adjust his or her schema. Will he or she feel shame or move away from shame to acceptance or pride? In one sense, this readjustment of sexual values and attitudes can go through similar identity stages, as proposed by Cass (1979). Sexuality does not remain static over the life span; as we grow and mature, the sexual continuum can be fluid, allowing for change of sexual expression.

Of course, as with most behaviors in general, sexual fantasy can also have negative associations, one being to commit sexual offenses, such as rape, exhibitionism, and child sexual abuse, but this begs the argument of whether people can control sexual urges. And as with other addictive behaviors, some people struggle with lack of impulse control. Additionally, sexual dysfunction can be affected by the lack of sexual fantasies or guilt about having sexual fantasies (Cado & Leitenberg, 1990).

Sexual Fantasy and Sexual Dysfunction

Hypoactive sexual desire disorder is a lack of sexual desire and one of the most common presenting complaints at sexual dysfunction clinics (Beck, 1995; Donahey & Carroll, 1993). According to the *Diagnostic and Statistical Manual of Mental Disorders* (American Psychiatric Association, 1994), a lack of sexual fantasies must be present for the diagnosis of hypoactive sexual desire disorder to be made. When considering the human sexual response cycle (desire, arousal, and orgasm), sexual fantasy is believed to precede sexual desire. So, lack of fantasies can contribute substantially to sexual dissatisfaction in relationships, both relational and recreational.

Sexual Fantasy and Sexual Health

Sexual fantasies that accompany masturbation include sexual activity with one's partner, same-sex sexual activity, reliving a past sexual experience, sex with an idealized partner, a romantic encounter, and oral sex and group sex, to name a few. Some argue that sexual fantasies reflect healthy sexuality and are simply another form of normal sexual stimulation used to promote sexual arousal and enjoyment (Singer, 1966). There are more questions than answers when it comes to explaining connections between healthy and unhealthy sexual functioning and behaviors, but the current body of existing literature provides ample documentation of continued research to aid in sex therapy and sex education. And with the onslaught and sheer abundance of social media, Internet access, advertising, and visual media, understanding how these connections relate to human sexual behavior are even more important today. Being able to sift through the maze of how sexual fantasies predict sexual behavior will also help us to better inform therapeutic treatment and interventions. So, what does all this have to do with addiction?

CONNECTIONS TO SUBSTANCE ABUSE

Sexual Enhancement

One reason why women with drinking problems and sexual dysfunction experience higher rates of relapse may be related to the fact that they use alcohol to try to increase sexual pleasure and/or reduce sexual distress (Wilsnack, 1991). In one study, participants were asked a series of questions regarding alcohol and sexual activity. Both alcoholic and treatment controls reported significant numbers that said that they felt less sexually inhibited when drinking (Beckman, 1979). They also believed that they desired, enjoyed, and engaged in sexual activities more when they were drinking (usually when drinking "a little" as opposed to "a lot").

More alcoholics (men and women) reported that a little drinking enhanced sexual desire and enjoyment as compared with controls. Among the participants studied, only 19 to 27 percent said that their sexual desire, enjoyment, and activity were greater without alcohol (Blume, 1991). The positive relationship between drinking levels and reported effects suggests that expectations of decreased sexual inhibition, enhanced sexual pleasure, and increased interpersonal closeness may be motives for heavier drinking in women (Wilsnack, 1991).

Sexual Dysfunction

In terms of sexual anatomy and functioning related to substance use, there are a number of issues that may influence a person's decision to use. A number of alcoholics have reported higher levels of sexual adjustment problems, including lack of sexual arousal, infrequent orgasm, impaired erection, ability to ejaculate, and decreased sexual interest (e.g., Covington & Kohen, 1984; Peugh & Belenko, 2001; Schaefer & Evans, 1987). The perceived effects of alcohol on sexual arousal and responsiveness compared to the actual physiological effects illustrate some interesting results as well; physiological responses are actually *diminished* over time with repeated use of alcohol and substances.

Expectancies

Many new substance users (or those who use infrequently) report an increased perception of sexual desire (the aphrodisiac) or belief that substances will enhance sexual pleasure. Some of these drugs include alcohol, methamphetamines, cocaine, and marijuana. Although commonly used drugs do not directly impact the arousal or orgasm stages, initial perceptions coupled with prolonged, heavy use over time can impact sexual health and inhibit sexual functioning. "With higher doses and long-term use, alcohol and drugs can impair sexual response, reduce sexual desire, and contribute to sexual dysfunction" (Peugh & Belenko, 2001, pp. 229–230). These authors also advocate for treatment providers to consider how the sexual problems of substance-abusing men and women are associated with the addiction and recovery process.

When we make the connections to sexual fantasy and desire, *the use of alcohol and other drugs is expected to enhance sexual outcomes*, whether a more intense orgasm or just the ability to be sexual. So, alcohol or substance use can become intrinsically linked to sexual fantasy and behaviors, making it a treatment issue. The following example provides some context:

> When I was younger, like I started watching pornos before I started having sex, so I noticed that I would watch the pornos to watch the girls and not the guys, and I always felt ashamed of that, wanting to have sex with girls. Until one day I was just drunk and just had sex with a girl and a guy, and I liked it. So if I knew I was gonna have a threesome with a girl and a guy, I'd just get drunk and high and go have fun and fill out my fantasies. That made me really comfortable.

Another client made the direct connection to the use of alcohol in order to be sexual with another person, also noting that he had more comfort in masturbating than having sex with his partner:

> My drinking years is when it [alcohol use] really impacted my sexual image. I can remember saying to my first wife, well, I remember feeling this way, that I had to get drunk before I could be intimate with her physically, and then I ended up telling her this, and I don't think there's anything that I could have said after that that would have made up for it, and everything went downhill after that, but that's the way I felt. I had to drink to have sex, and then later on I had to drink to do a lot of things, but I think I felt inadequate or I felt that I couldn't be fully engaged in it, that I had to maybe be buzzed or escape in order to enjoy sex with someone else 'cause during masturbation it didn't bother me or whatever, but it was sex with a partner. And it happened on occasion with people when I was not married, so it was, it happened, it was not just her; it was in other people, and it was pretty much just the sexual, the act of sex, that I had to be that way. I still felt caring and intimate and all these other things on a normal basis, but it's like I had, it was part of a ritual. I had to drink before I had sex; it was a ritual.

Both of these individuals make the connection of feeling ashamed about fantasizing or engaging in recreational sex, and their coping mechanisms involved drinking to lower inhibitions in order to be sexual (the man) or engage in the "taboo" behavior (in the first example).

Internalizing Negative Perceptions: One Client's Experience

When working with clients concerning their feelings of shame or guilt over sexual pleasure and past behaviors, we need to explore the origins of the beliefs so as to begin a process of validating, then reversing negative perceptions they hold of themselves. Recreational sex is perfectly normal, but understanding the connections to substance use are lost if the provider believes that the behavior is "bad" or "sinful" or, worse, condemns the client and prematurely labels him or her as a sexual addict or as deviant. Making this mistake can negatively impact the trajectory of successful treatment planning. We need to be careful not to impose our personal bias and value judgments on clients.

With regard to the treatment process, other effects of how internalized feelings of shame attached to nonprocreative sex were common themes that arose in clients' stories:

> Okay, what I learned about sexuality growing up is that, it was part of life, it was part of something that we do. I was taught that for Genesis in the Bible that God created Adam and Eve so that we could procreate and bring about more people, so, therefore, and unfortunately I had a mom who was not very caring, so I always wanted that touch and hugging, and I found it in men. God rest his soul, my father is deceased, he was murdered, but it caused confusion about how I feel about that whole situation because it was a bad thing for him to do [incest], but in the other sense that it struck this thing in me where I think I'm addicted to sex. I enjoy sex. Not that I'm sleeping with anybody and everybody, but I, like, I do have a partner whether it's male or female. I have a pretty healthy sex life with them. I'm not shy at all about with my body. I'm an ex-prostitute, I used to dance, and so it's something that I enjoy doing, sex, I live it so.

This particular client has confusion over her strong connection to sexual pleasure, which is not bad; her religious messages are more than likely what caused her conflict with wanting to enjoy sex but being raised to believe that sex was only for procreation within a marriage. Her recreational sexual activities were internalized as being bad. It is erroneous thinking to believe that the enjoyment of sex equates to being addicted to it. From what she shared, her recent sexual behaviors did not involve indiscriminate acts, merely behaviors that are stigmatized in our society (dancing and prostitution).

Reversing Negative Messages

Avenues for exploration with this particular case should include discussions about healthy sexuality, sexual pleasure, and normalization of recreational sex. We could also help her connect some of her past behaviors to substance use and explore whether she used substances to cover up resulting shame from her dancing and prostitution. I would also explore the topic of masturbation and fantasy in the context of how to satiate her sex drive in recovery. Triggers from sexual pleasure in addiction could be explored as well in order to begin a relapse prevention plan. Most of all, I would work with her to help her feel proud of her body and good about her connection to pleasure instead of shame. It is our responsibility to help clients reverse the negative messages they may have internalized regarding sex and sexuality.

MASTURBATION AND SEXUAL HEALTH

In his essay on "masturbation as a means of achieving sexual health," Eli Coleman explains that masturbation takes on the power of a meaning within individual and society; these can be both positive and negative and are often determined by the interaction between prevailing societal attitudes and individual attitudes and behavior:

The Negative Power. Because of the stigma promoted by cultural and religious beliefs, masturbation has the power to create intense guilt and shame in individuals. It can also cause conflicts in relationships. This can lead to further problems, such as mental and sexual disorder. Because of the stigma of masturbation promoted by many of the world's religions, this can contribute to spiritual alienation as well.

The Positive Power. Masturbation gives the individual the opportunity to learn about his or her body and sexual response. Because sexual pleasure is given to oneself, it has been speculated that it contributes to an individual's sense of ownership, control, and autonomy over his or her own body. Bodily integrity is not only a sexual right but also a key ingredient in sexual health (Coleman, 2002; World Association for Sexology, 1999).

Positive Attributes of Masturbation

Positive attributes of masturbation are that it increases orgasmic capacity, provides satisfaction in relationships, relieves the pressure to be sexual in relationships, provides safe alternatives to risky sexual behaviors, provides a means of increasing comfort with one's own body and self-esteem, decreases anxiety in sexual contexts, and provides a sexual outlet when a partner is unavailable or disinterested in sex (reducing seeking sex elsewhere), to name a few. Sex therapists have long utilized masturbatory techniques to help treat sexual dysfunctions with great success rates, as learning about sexual response can be practiced alone. Masturbation is being viewed more as a critical ingredient for establishing improved self-identity and self-esteem and improving intimacy as well as a pathway to increasing one's sexual comfort, satisfaction, and overall health.

Promoting Positive Sexual Self-Image with Masturbation

In terms of promoting positive sexual self-image with regard to masturbation, counselors should consider how to incorporate ways in which discussions can be facilitated. The media can provide avenues for healthy discussion. For example, in the television series *Homeland*, the main character, who had been rescued after eight years in captivity in the Middle East, is integrating back into his life in the United States. His first sexual experience with his wife in an early episode resembled that of a rape scene. Following that episode, he begins sleeping on the floor because he is experiencing violent flashbacks. One night, his wife climbs out of bed and on the floor with him and attempts to open the door to discussion of "catching up" on changes since he was presumed dead (she was having a sexual relationship with the husband's best friend when they discovered him alive overseas). She then proceeds to make sexual advances, to which he responds by pushing her away, taking her negligee off, and masturbating to orgasm while viewing her; her eyes are averted from him during this scene, and neither one of them discusses it afterward.

Considering how masturbation can cause problems within relationships because of how it may be viewed, this is a perfect example of how a follow-up group or part of a group on masturbation and fantasy might be facilitated. Taping an excerpt of movies and shows with educational and relevant content can provide ample opportunities for rich discussion of sexuality topics for use within the treatment setting. People masturbate for many reasons, and within stable, committed relationships, the practice of masturbation may create tension or a threat, depending on the relationship dynamics. It may also be used to enhance sexual pleasure and to incorporate sexual variety. Being able to openly discuss what some of these conflicts are and why they exist can help individuals learn how to communicate within a relationship as well as discover new ways to enhance sexual pleasure. In the treatment setting, providing safe alternatives for risky behavior or relapse triggers related to sexual behaviors, this is critical.

Broaching sensitive topics that are perceived as deviant can be risky in and of themselves, depending on the personal values of each partner within a relationship. Many committed partners have never discussed the full continuum of sexual behaviors; and this impacts communication. Having an environment in which these conversations can take place can help clients develop comfort around sexual communication. When we examine the roles that masturbation can take in promoting positive sexual health, especially by helping a person reclaim a sense of control over his or her body, we can start to make connections between helping those who have been abused to regain a sense of power in their lives.

SUGGESTED ACTIVITY

The following activity is recommended for both clients and providers.
Goal: To normalize competing sexual views (procreative, relational, and recreational) and acknowledge the continuum of relationships that exist in societies.
Rationale: In terms of related "taboo" sexual behaviors that are historically stigmatized, a discussion of relational issues in the treatment setting is warranted in order to normalize the different relational arrangements, types of behaviors one might engage in with regard to their situation, and how these are linked to fantasy, sexual pleasure, and masturbation. This activity legitimizes, for many, the variety of relationships they may have had in their addiction and opens the door for future exploration of a variety of sexual topics. Providing opportunities for participants to reassess their attitudes toward different sexual lifestyles will help reduce anxiety and promote discussion of sexual behaviors within relationships.

Time: 90 minutes
Objectives: Participants will do the following:

- List six different relationships that exist in society
- Distinguish between procreative, relational, and recreational sex
- Identify personal causes of shame associated with the three views of sex

- Identify personal connections between substance use and sexual behavior
- Create a personal view of sex that is positive

Materials:

- Eleven sheets of newsprint, each with the following labels: "traditional monogamy," "chaste monogamy," "child-free marriage," "group marriage" (threesomes, foursomes, moresomes, and so on), "swinging/group sex," "single parenthood," "open marriage/committed relationship," "secret affair," "communal living," "lifelong celebration/chastity," "serial monogamy"
- Masking tape
- Markers

Spectrum of Relationships (about 45 to 50 minutes):

1. Newsprint should be taped on walls, with the bottom half taped up so that each title cannot be viewed.
2. Facilitator introduces the topic "Competing views of sexuality" and describes some goals associated with the topic (ideally, this should tie in from a previous lesson; following a sensitive issues lesson would be appropriate).
3. Break the group into pairs. Ask each pair to stand in front of one of the newsprint, untape it, and then spend a few minutes discussing and writing down personal reactions to the relationships. If they are not sure what each area is, explain briefly in order to keep the activity moving; ask them not to censor their thoughts.
4. After about two to three minutes, ask each pair to rotate one sheet to their right. Pairs should repeat this process until each pair has visited each sheet once.
5. Ask the group to take their original seats and process with the following questions:
   - What was it like for you to do this activity?
   - What feelings came up for you as you moved around the room and viewed what other people thought of certain types of relationships?
   - How might your feelings about the material be connected to your addiction?
   - Was anything about this activity surprising for you? Why?

- How will this information help you in your recovery? (For providers, how will this help you in your work with clients?)

6. Facilitator must be prepared to field emotional reactions, negative comments, and potential dissension in group responses. Explanations of the relationships and how they are manifest in society will begin to tie in concepts from earlier topics, such as lesbian, gay, bisexual, and transgender issues; reproductive bias; sexually transmitted diseases/HIV; values clarification; intimacy; nonconsensual sex; the right to sexual freedom; masturbation; marriage; infidelity; communication; secrecy; and other issues. Being able to tie in what surfaces in a positive manner is critical, making sure that tolerance of others' relational choices is promoted and respected.

The Competing Views of Sexuality (30–40 minutes):

1. A brief overview of the three competing views of sexuality should now be presented, followed by some small-group work.
2. Break the group into three smaller groups. Each group should have one of the competing views as their topic.
3. Groups should discuss these questions: (1) What are the positive and negative aspects of your assigned view? (2) How has your assigned view harmed yourself or another? (3) How might your assigned view affect someone in recovery or active addiction? (4) What can you do in terms of reversing any negative messages?
4. Homework could involve having participants create a personal view of sexual fantasy/masturbation and relationships that is positive.

NEXT STEPS

Finding meaningful ways to introduce sexual content can be complicated and intimidating. I hope the information presented in this chapter will help you begin to understand how the historical views on masturbation and competing views of sexual behaviors impact how we view the sexual behaviors of clients in treatment and our reactions to them. The activities can provide the impetus for opening the door for honest communication regarding masturbation, fantasy, and the origins of shameful irrational beliefs. Recognizing the links between harmful and shaming messages regarding sexuality in all its forms should be explored in a sexual health group. I have successfully utilized these activities with clients, students, and providers. Many people have never broached certain topics, and even if all participants are not actively engaged in the discussions, being exposed to the material will get them thinking about what their personal values are and how well the values fit (or don't) in their lives. Too many people experience guilt and shame over their sexuality because they perceive that they deviate from the expected societal norm, especially substance-abusing clients. The importance of including discussions on masturbation, sexual fantasy, and other relational arrangements are critical to reverse negative learning and illustrate the diversity within human sexual relationships.

RESOURCES

Books

Joannides, P. N. (2011). *The guide to getting it on!* Waldport, OR: Goofy Foot Press.

Stenger, J., & Van Neck, A. (2001). *Masturbation: The history of a great terror*. New York: Palgrave.

Waxman, J. (2007). *Getting off: A woman's guide to masturbation*. Berkeley, CA: Seal Press.

Online Resources

Sex Information Online. http://dodsonandross.com/topic/masturbation?page=1.

Sexual Med. http://www.sexualmed.org/index.cfm/sexual-health-resources/articles/fantasy-and-orgasm.

NINE

Good Sex!

We settle for so-so sex because most of us don't know how sexual we could be; we know only how sexual we are. How sexual we are has been shaped by decades of indoctrination by . . . family and friends, teachers, religious leaders, and romantic partners, not to mention a society that worships a bewildering fusion of childlike sexual innocence and cynical, nihilistic hedonism. . . . So what is normal? It all depends on what's normal for you.

—Clayton and Cantor-Cooke (2007)

What is good sex? Is it having a satisfying orgasm with a partner? Is it engaging in frequent sexual interactions or perhaps making a new connection with a potential partner that feels healthy and makes us happy about possibilities? Is good sex having that sexual experience where we can tell our partner what pleases us and can ask our partner what pleases him or her and then be able to reciprocate? Or is good sex feeling good about ourselves as sexual beings whether we are "doing it" or not? I maintain that it can be all of the above and more. Hopefully by now, you are thinking about sexuality in a broader sense and integrating the subtleties of sex into your psyche. Good sex is a tapestry of feelings, experiences, and attitudes woven together in a unique pattern of color and texture. Good sex is a combination of sexual health and self-care that includes many facets of Sexual Beingness. Good sex is coming to the center of ourselves and not feeling ashamed of who we are as sexual beings.

There are many books out there dealing specifically with sexual pleasure and relationships, some of which have already been provided in the resource sections. Although sexual pleasure will be discussed in terms of good sex, a holistic approach to sexual health is explored in this chapter. Good sex is about being empowered to take our sexual rights and be happy in the world. Core beliefs will be explored, as will fostering sexual health through positive sexual self-esteem and empowerment.

DECLARATION OF SEXUAL RIGHTS

In 1978, a global organization formed to promote sexual health and sexual rights and to further the understanding and development of sexology throughout the world. The World Association for Sexology (WAS) has worked with health care providers, sexuality educators, researchers, and policymakers to endorse position statements condemning sexual torture, discrimination and bias, the genital mutilation of women, and more. In 1994, WAS adopted a declaration of sexual rights. The declaration views sexual health as a fundamental right based on the inherent freedom, dignity, and equality of all human beings. In order for human beings to develop a healthy sexuality, these rights must be recognized, promoted, respected, and defended by all societies through all means. WAS also developed a millennium document that specifies and elaborates on eight distinct aspects of sexual health that play a part in fostering human development; the full document is 171 pages and is included in the resource section of this chapter. In order to promote sexual health for everyone, these documents address many of the most complicated and urgent social problems of our current time.

The WAS declaration of sexual rights includes the following:

1. The right to sexual freedom. Sexual freedom encompasses the possibility for individuals to express their full sexual potential. However, this excludes all forms of sexual coercion, exploitation and abuse at any time and situations in life.

2. The right to sexual autonomy, sexual integrity, and safety of the sexual body. This right involves the ability to make autonomous decisions about one's sexual life within a context of one's own personal and social ethics. Its also encompasses control and enjoyment of our own bodies free from torture, mutilation and violence of any sort.

3. The right to sexual privacy. This involves the right for individual decision and behaviors about intimacy as long as they do not intrude on the sexual rights of others.

4. The right to sexual equity. This refers to freedom from all forms of discrimination regardless of sex, gender, sexual orientation, age, race, social class, religion, or physical and emotional disability.

5. The right to sexual pleasure. Sexual pleasure, including autoeroticism, is a source of physical, psychological, intellectual and spiritual well being.

6. The right to emotional sexual expression. Sexual expression is more than erotic pleasure or sexual acts. Individuals have a right to express their sexuality through communication, touch, emotional expression and love.

7. The right to sexually associate freely. This means the possibility to marry or not, to divorce, and to establish other types of responsible sexual associations.

8. The right to make free and responsible reproductive choices. This encompasses the right to decide whether or not to have children, the number and spacing of children, and the right to full access to the means of fertility regulation.

9. The right to sexual information based upon scientific inquiry. This right implies that sexual information should be generated through the process of unencumbered and yet scientifically ethical inquiry, and disseminated in appropriate ways at all societal levels.

10. The right to comprehensive sexuality education. This is a lifelong process from birth throughout the lifecycle and should involve all social institutions.

11. The right to sexual health care. Sexual health care should be available for prevention and treatment of all sexual concerns, problems and disorders. (http://www.worldsexology.org/resources)

Even as we move forward in the twenty-first century, learning positive messages about sexuality growing up is not the accepted norm. The secrecy, ignorance, and trauma surrounding sex continue to prevail, and a positive sexual self-image comes slowly, if at all, for people as they mature. Living in an age of media-based information brings a new set of challenges. We are bombarded with images of a sexual nature through television, movies, the Internet, and technology. Access to sexual information is literally at our fingertips, so having the knowledge of how to assess accuracy, relevance, and meaning of these data for us and our families is critical. Because certain aspects of sexuality are so charged with negative affect, many websites reflect values of intolerance and hatred toward sexual issues.

It is our responsibility to familiarize ourselves with sexual media that supports tolerance and sex-positive messages. We don't want to fall into the trap of letting someone's morality jade our ability to take the judgment out of working with people whose sexual behaviors and values we do not share. After all, this isn't about us; it's about the people we are trying to help recover. Most of them have already experienced more than their share of stigma and its psychological consequences.

BENEFITS OF SEXUAL HEALTH

Consistently in societies, sexual health is viewed from the negative consequences of sexual health, many of which have already been discussed in this text. These include effects of sexual abuse and assault, sexually transmitted infections/HIV, unwanted pregnancy, rape, incest, out-of-control sexual behaviors, and sexual dysfunction. As we begin to reframe how we view sexuality, it is important to begin to examine the positive effects of sexual healthy expression. A white paper on the health benefits of sexual expression was published in cooperation between the Planned Parenthood Federation of America (2003) and the Society for the Scientific Study of Sexuality. This paper outlined some of the numerous positive health benefits from research associated with sexual expression; these expressions included higher levels of sexual activities, orgasm, and masturbation, some of which are listed here:

- *Longevity*—Several studies with large sample sizes found positive associations between frequency of sexual intercourse, frequency of orgasm, and enjoyment of intercourse and living longer (Davey Smith, Frankel, & Yarnell, 1997; Palmore, 1982; Persson, 1981).
- *Heart disease and stroke*—Studies that examined frequent sexual intercourse, orgasm, sex hormones in men found links to decreased risk for stroke heart attack (Booth, Johnson, & Granger, 1999; Ebrahim, May, McCarron, Frankel, & Davey, 2002; Fogari et al., 2002).
- *Breast cancer*—Hormones associated with sexual arousal and orgasm have been suggested to decrease the risk of cancer (Lê, Bacheloti, & Hill, 1989; Petridou, Giokas, Mucci, & Trichopoulos, 2000).
- *Immunity*—Sexual activity and orgasm may bolster the immune system in men and women through sleep (endorphins released from orgasm facilitate sleep), youthfulness (frequency of sexual activity), and fitness (frequent sex is associated with better health habits and burning calories and fat) (Charnetski & Brennan, 2001; Ellison, 2000; Weeks & James, 1998).

- *Sexual and reproductive health*—Relationships between sexual behavior and orgasm have been found to reduce the incidence of endometriosis, enhance fertility (both men and women), regulate the menstrual cycle, relieve menstrual cramps, and prevent preterm delivery in pregnancies (Cutler, 1991; Ellison, 2000; Levin, 2002; Meaddough, Olive, Gallup, Perlin, & Kliman, 2002; Sayle et al., 2002).
- *Pain management*—Physiological responses associated with sexual activity have been shown to reduce chronic pain, and sex hormones reduce pain associated with arthritis, menstrual cramps, migraines, and other conditions (e.g., Ellison, 2000; Komisaruk & Whipple, 1995).
- *Psychological, emotional, social, and spiritual health*—A growing body of research demonstrates that sexual expression can improve quality of life and self-esteem, reduce stress, reduce depression and risk for suicide, increase intimacy between partners, and increase spirituality (e.g., Bagley & Tremblay, 1997; Coleman, 2002; Ellison, 2000; Hurlbert & Whittaker, 1991; Laumann, Gagnon, Michael, & Michaels, 1998; Ogden, 2001; Weeks, 2002; Zamboni & Crawford, 2002).

These links clearly need to be considered when we are working with the sexuality issues of substance abusers to help them recognize the health benefits and develop ways in which to incorporate a healthy sense of sexuality into the recovery process. This requires providers to also develop their own sense of a positive framework of sexuality in order to provide effective avenues for their clients' sexual health. Focusing on the positives rather than the negatives will enable us to make the shift in mind-set from pathology to health.

SEXUAL SELF-ESTEEM AS A MEASURE FOR SEXUAL HEALTH?

How we perceive ourselves has a great impact on whether we take care of ourselves, how we value who we are, and if we feel we are worthy of being happy. With regard to sexual health, a positive self-image is integral to the process of attaining balance in good sex. I propose that by incorporating the concept of sexual self-esteem as a measure for certain aspects of sexual health, we can begin to assess and address sexuality in the treatment realm.

The terms "sexual self-concept" and "sexual self-esteem" have often been used interchangeably and defined similarly. Some definitions of sexual self-concept include "the view of the self as a sexual being in terms of attractiveness, desirability, and self-worth" and an "individual's evaluation of his or her own feelings and actions" (Jorgenson, 1983; Winter, 1988). One definition of sexual self-esteem is "the tendency to value, versus devalue, one's own sexuality, thereby being able to approach rather than avoid sexual experiences both with self and others" (Gaynor & Underwood, 1995). Sexual self-esteem is described as a learned combination of values and experiences based on the interaction between sexual values learned in the family; peer group values regarding bodily appearance, dress, mannerisms, sexual orientation, and gender; and both positive and negative personal sexual experiences. All these concepts touch on components included in the definition of sexual health.

The construct of sexual self-esteem is still being researched and explored, so definitions of this concept are not consistent. Several instruments have been developed to measure sexual self-esteem in people. The sexual esteem subscale, which has been used most frequently (Snell & Papini, 1989), is limited by its narrow definition of sexual self-esteem, which concerns only a person's ability to relate sexually to another person. Lacking in this definition and measure are components that correspond to previous definitions of self-esteem, such as virtue and power. More specific domains of sexual self-esteem are measured in other instruments.

Gaynor and Underwood's (1995) construct of sexual self-esteem is rather broad, measuring behaviors, values, and needs. Optimal sexuality is viewed as including reciprocal pleasure and exchange, with the ideal development proceeding from self to partner context. One problem with this measure is that it appears to neglect a positive view of sexual development for individuals who choose not to engage in sexual behaviors with a partner.

A more comprehensive view defines sexual self-esteem as "one's affective reactions to one's sexual thoughts, feelings and behaviors" (Zeanah & Schwarz, 1996). This measure is appealing for a broader scope of the population since sexuality is given a relatively liberal definition. This scale does not discriminate between individuals who have engaged in sexual activity and those who have not. Sexual behavior includes a variety of behaviors, and this is inclusive for those individuals who are currently involved in relationships that may or may not include sexual intercourse as well as inclusion of other sexual behaviors and experiences. This measure has also been used with samples of women and men with similar results.

Results from numerous studies utilizing this scale have consistently found low sexual self-esteem scores from participants who have experienced forms of child and adult sexual abuse, rape, incest, and assault in both clinical (having mental health or other psychological issues) and nonclinical (mainstream society) samples. Low sexual self-esteem relates to feeling negatively about one's sexual experiences and perceptions. High sexual self-esteem equates with having positive perception of one's sexual self.

Interesting findings from some of the research on sexual self-esteem might fly in the face of what practitioners may have traditionally asked of their clients. Several studies found positive sexual self-esteem in participants who engaged in greater sexual activities; the more experience they had, the higher their sexual self-esteem (i.e., Seal, Minichiello & Omodei 1997; Shapiro & Schwarz, 1997; Zeanah & Schwarz, 1996). Recovering participants in relationships versus those clients not in relationships had higher sexual self-esteem as well (James, 2011). So, being in a relationship in early recovery *can* be a healthy component for clients. Our society values people who are in relationships, particularly women, so the need to establish or continue romantic relationships makes them feel normal and accepted by their peers.

One of the subscales on the revised sexual self-esteem scale that I developed measures sexual satisfaction. Individuals scoring low in this area are not likely to be having the "good sex" feelings we would like them to. The following are the questions from the sexual satisfaction subscale: (1) I am happy about my sex life; (2) All in all, I feel satisfied with my sex life; (3) I feel disappointed with my sex life (reverse scored item); (4) I am where I want to be sexually, at this point in my life; (5) I feel good about the place of sex in my life; and (6) I wish things were different for me sexually (reverse scored). This subscale can be used to measure high or low sexual self-esteem in the area of "good" sex. And for those clients who may have low sexual self-esteem, having a way to measure improvement can help providers track client progress and the outcomes of a sexual health program.

CORE BELIEFS

A number of components go into how we view ourselves, including the beliefs we have learned on life's journey. We learn these beliefs through things such as our environments, families, spiritual affiliations, peers, and interactions with others. And, depending on the nature of the learning, we also begin a process of internalizing these beliefs as we move through the life span. Of course, early development sets the framework for learning and tends to be the most influential.

Most societies throughout the span of time have held men and women to different standards regarding both sexual behavior and drinking behavior. Perceptions of women violating traditional norms regarding sexual behavior have been associated with the violation of drinking norms, that is, heavier drinking by women (Wilsnack, 1991). The results are stereotypes of drinking women as more promiscuous, more sexually responsive, and more vulnerable to sexual advances.

The boundary of what is considered acceptable and unacceptable behavior for men and women begins with early childhood socialization. Whereas traditionally boys have been encouraged to be aggressive, physically combative, independent, nonemotional, and outward oriented, girls are more often taught to be passive, dependent, emotional, and relationship oriented (Miller, 1986). Men are taught to act knowledgeable about sex, to be comfortable with their bodies, and to unconsciously touch themselves and their genitals. As the sexual initiators, men are also expected to know all about sex before marriage (Harrison & Pennel, 1989; Richmond-Abbot 1983). Men are also expected to be assertive in physical relationships, the ones who seek out and choose a sexual partner, initiate sexual behavior, and orchestrate the sexual encounter.

Women, on the other hand, are discouraged from learning about sex, touching or thinking about their genitals, or being sexually assertive (Schaffer, 1981). Many women can't even speak about the sexual anatomy without using such euphemisms as "down there" and have never looked at their genitals. They are socialized toward passivity in their intimate relationships, such as waiting to be approached by the other person. Women's sexual signaling must be somewhat subtle, for if she is too assertive, she may be labeled as "easy," or "loose," and possibly sexually abused. The disdain and punishment attributed to sexually assertive women disconnects them from their sexual feelings. This is also exacerbated by the expectation that women will orient their behavior toward the satisfaction of their partner. Many women have spent so many years trying to please their partner that they have no awareness of what their own needs are (Covington, 1991).

Stigma is the main psychological issue differentiating the substance abuse of females from that of males (Covington, 2002). Although drinking is viewed more positively for men, women who drink are viewed more harshly by society, as there is conflict between femininity and the roles of wife and mother. The terms "lush," "slut," and "bad mother" are often associated with female addicts. Women often internalize the stigma from these labels and feel shame, despair, fear, and guilt when they are suffering from addictions to drugs and/or alcohol (Covington, 2002). The constant threat of consequences and stigma is stressful over time. As a result, women will typically deny or minimize the extent of their substance use. These feelings of embarrassment and shame were a common theme among participants from both their substance use and their sexual experiences:

- "I always felt ashamed of that, wanting to have sex with girls [female client]."
- "Prostituting myself, I had got raped by three guys at once, and I don't even know any of them, and after that it was just like, I felt like a whore."
- "I don't like to think about that stuff; it's embarrassing, and it's not me, and if somebody brings it up to me, I don't even want to talk about it, I get really embarrassed."
- "I don't like to have to think about what I did and what occurred and the people that I hurt because then it just makes me feel like less of a person."
- "I kept my body numb, so I didn't feel the pain of being, you know, depressed all the time, but it stayed there because it made my addiction get worse, made me get worse as a person, physically, mentally, and emotionally. I put myself down and allowed others to put me down. It just made my addiction worse."
- "The nurse told me that . . . and that I was a wild child and that I probably deserved it [being raped] or provided it or whatever. But I remember, *me* feeling guilty and ashamed of myself in the end."

The internalization of these beliefs contributes to low sexual self-esteem in more than one area. One of the components of shame is the internalized feeling of being morally deficient. It is one matter to know that some of our behaviors can be labeled as bad; this typically results in someone feeling guilty. But when that guilt seeps into our psyche and we internalize it, we begin to feel as if *we* are bad, and this can result in the experience of shame. Shame is more difficult to treat, as it relates to how we view ourselves rather than our behaviors. It is easier to change behavior than something that we feel we have no control over, in this case, ourselves as being bad. And the labels our clients wear—addict, drug user, dope fiend, slut, whore, sexual abuser, sex addict, prostitute, and so on—all carry great stigma and can lead to feelings of shame and low self-worth. So, in order to reverse the negative impact these core beliefs have on the psyche, we need to develop a new schema for clients to view themselves in.

EMPOWERMENT

What can we do to foster positive sexual self-esteem and develop positive core beliefs in our clients? First of all, we have to believe that positive sexual self-image equates, in part, to experiencing a healthy sexuality. When people are comfortable with their sexuality, when they know what is pleasurable to them and are able to negotiate pleasure with their partner, they are more likely to be satisfied and to take less sexual risk.

Good sex includes being able to experiment safely and appropriately, set sexual boundaries, negotiate pleasure with a partner, feel sexually competent in sexual situations, know their own preferences, and feel good about being able to please their sexual partner as well. "A developmental approach to sexual health over the lifespan recognizes the reality that all human beings need to be able to explore their sexuality in order to develop and nurture who they are" (Robinson, Bockting, Rosser, Miner, & Coleman, 2002). For those who have not had this healthy sexual development (substance abusers in particular), we are in an excellent position to foster this process in treatment and recovery.

A cornerstone philosophy for many AIDS organizations utilizes the construct of empowerment. Empowerment includes being able to foster positive self-efficacy in oneself and/or others. In the HIV realm, initial diagnosis is usually devastating; it is the ultimate lack of power, having an illness that may eventually claim your life. That being said, there are many cofactors to health, both negative and positive. One of the things I was able to do with my HIV clients was to teach them about these cofactors and help them to incorporate positive change into their lives. This, coupled with a belief that they could beat this disease or stay healthy, often resulted in better health outcomes. My clients who were pessimistic and negative attracted similarly negative health outcomes.

Living with a substance use problem has a similar trajectory, with similar cofactors that can affect a person's ability to live a healthy, happy existence. Being able to embrace a philosophy that empowers clients rather than one that continues to browbeat them for making mistakes is the best place to start. Take the following story, for example. I once had a client who was infected with HIV through his injection drug–using behaviors. He was from a large urban area and had relocated to a smaller city in his attempts to recover. When I first took my job at the agency, pretty much everyone rolled their eyes when his name was mentioned in department meetings for case conferences, or in the hallways. He was your typical "resistant," "noncompliant" client.

The first time we met face-to-face was in jail. "Ralph," as I will refer to him as, was in and out of jail because of consequences from his drug-using behaviors. He was a very funny and likable guy. Over the months and years, we built an alliance that was strong. I continued looked for his strengths in our interactions (keeping an apartment when he was in jail, attempts at recovery, good sense of humor, and ability to get his needs met) rather than always focusing on his weaknesses. I found that this concept was alien to Ralph, and occasionally he would comment to me, saying that no one in his life had ever had anything positive to say about him. No matter what happened, when Ralph came back for services, I was there, encouraging him but letting him make his choices and live with the outcomes. I also wasn't afraid to call him out on his behaviors, and he usually laughed when I did, then we talked about what he was really dealing with. I think he appreciated my honesty. In addition, we had collaborated in our process.

Collaboration requires us to acknowledge our responsibility to our clients while deferring to their personal expertise and authority. Ralph was the expert in his life, and I allowed him to exercise control in his decision making regardless of the results. In other words, he benefited the most in the end because he had the power over his own process; I operated as a facilitator and a recovery coach.

Eventually, Ralph moved to another part of the state, and we lost contact, as I had taken another position within the agency. One day, at a staff meeting, our volunteer coordinator had returned from a conference at the state capitol and announced that she had seen Ralph at the conference. Apparently, he had been clean and sober for a couple of years and told her that if it weren't for me, he never would have made it. Of course, I was flattered (and in tears from the happy news) but said that Ralph is the one who did it; I merely helped empower him to believe in himself.

One of the more frustrating concepts of using an empowerment approach is that we have no control over the outcomes. Our job is to plant the seeds and foster their growth. We foster their growth by *watering the seeds, not the weeds*. This is at the heart of the matter. Ralph knew all the bad things about himself; he had heard them all his life. He needed someone to tell him that he had good characteristics and positive attributes. He needed someone to believe in him and show him how. He needed someone not to give up on him when he gave up on himself. He needed someone to be there when he came back and not judge him for all he did wrong. It sounds simplistic, but it is not. Letting someone have their process and for us to let go of the outcomes is challenging. That means that we, as providers, need to be able to conceptualize and measure change

Figure 9.1   Shifting to Positive Language.

Reframing Labels and Perceptions

Chronic	←————————→	Resilient
Non-Compliant	←————————→	Independent
Resistant	←————————→	Cautious
Manipulative	←————————→	Skillful
Demanding	←————————→	Assertive
Frustrating	←————————→	Challenging
Not Ready	←————————→	Precontemplative

differently. We also need to be able to reframe our own negative perceptions into positive ones. This reframed perception can enable us to approach the client in a more positive manner (see Figure 9.1).

STAGING CLIENTS

Remember the stages of change model? Moving a client through the stages gives us an incremental method of measuring small changes in clients' growth. And measuring growth in more than one area is critical to fostering growth in other areas. For example, I staged Ralph in his housing, substance use, health, medication adherence, vocational efforts, and more. So, while he might have been contemplative or precontemplative about his substance use, he was in maintenance with his housing or medication adherence. This gave me other avenues to empower him with because when he was doing poorly with his recovery efforts, he was doing well in other areas, and I was able to focus on those successes to foster his belief that he was at least doing some things well. This may also seem simplistic, but for the client who has been told all of his or her life that he or she will never amount to anything, being treated with dignity and given hope are major collaborative tools for building self-efficacy.

TRUST

The therapeutic alliance is one of the most important tools you have. If you do not have the trust of your clients, you have no foundation on which to build. A counselor's interaction can be therapeutic whether your contact is one time or long term, frequent, or intermittent. Without this alliance, techniques will not work. The importance of an alliance is that it contradicts assumptions about past negative experiences a client has had, it provides a secure base from which to proceed, and it decreases a sense of isolation that is often experienced in addiction.

SUPPORT SERVICES

Of course, some of you are probably thinking right now that your agency does not provide these types of services, and how can you do all this work yourself? Another concept, recovery coaching, is discussed in the final chapter. While relatively new, this idea has existed to some degree unofficially as the "sponsor" in 12-step facilitation. While a sponsor and a recovery coach have different tasks and abilities, the idea of a positive long-term relationship with recovering people helps to keep them on track and have that support.

FACILITATING CHANGE

The story of Ralph and his journey serve to illustrate how empowerment concepts work in treatment on a basic level. Training on empowerment is also recommended for learning how to practice the skills. To a certain degree, personality type will have an impact on whether a counselor will have success with integrating this concept into their practices. If you are someone who always has to be in control, are not good at living with ambiguity, or are inflexible in approach, you may struggle more with being okay with the process. Empowerment is a process, as is recovery, and we need to be patient not only with the client but with ourselves as well.

In terms of good sex, one place to start with clients is to have them be able to identify what those negative core beliefs are that they have about themselves as sexual beings. This can be done through activities and homework in a sexual health group in recovery. Once these are identified, we have a starting place for change. Change starts inside our minds way before we ever decide to externalize the process to behaviors. And in the case of good sex, the results can take many different forms, including increased desire, better sexual functioning, ability to orgasm, the ability to have sober sex, and more.

PLISSIT MODEL

In addition to reframing core beliefs and empowering our clients to take charge of their sexual health, another area that can help them to improve sexual functioning is a therapeutic framework called "PLISSIT," an acronym for a four-step model of education and intervention. The PLISSIT model—Permission (P), Limited Information (LI), Specific Suggestions (SS), and Intensive Therapy (IT)—is one of the most commonly used and effective models for the assessment and intervention of sexual problems. The model follows a vertical structure, requiring greater knowledge and training as one moves up each level. It can also be used across cultural groups, as its format is flexible and adaptable.

Permission

This step involves asking permission of a client to speak about issues related to sex. Asking permission empowers clients by giving them control over whether they wish to pursue an area of sexuality. Permission can be implemented in numerous phases (e.g., individual therapy, a group session, intake, and so on) where sexual content needs to be discussed or is brought up by the client in a specific context. This stage validates sexuality as a legitimate concern and helps to form the therapeutic alliance.

Limited Information

This stage involves providing accurate information regarding the concern and dispelling false or unrealistic expectations, which can help alleviate feelings of guilt or anxiety. Enough information should be provided to help improve the sexual issue. Pamphlets, books, or videos may be provided for further education.

Specific Suggestions

In this stage, specific steps, instructions, and guidelines are provided to address specific problems and are tailored to each individual. Greater knowledge and expertise are required on the counselor's part. For example, if a client is still having trouble reestablishing intimacy within a relationship, more specific sexual counseling should take place; some of these could include the use of sensate focus activities.

Intensive Therapy

The final step (which the majority of clients do not reach) usually refers to conditions that require treatment by a physician, specialist, or therapist; for example, if erectile dysfunction believed to be associated with alcohol use does not improve over time, a medical referral related to the condition may be necessary in conjunction with other counseling.

Overall, the PLISSIT model provides a comprehensive plan to educate clients and treat a variety of sexual problems without needing to resort to intensive psychotherapy. Some of these have already been discussed in other chapters; this model frames sexual health education in a communication framework.

Client Experiences

In some of our interviews with clients, we asked them what things they think could help them with regard to sexual health in recovery. Not surprisingly, the responses related to components of promoting sexual health that were presented in this chapter. The following are a few selected comments:

Maria: A lot of us women, when we're early in recovery, our self-esteem is fairly low or artificially inflated, which is kind of that same thing but different. You know how do I learn how to become, or how to believe that I am worth waiting for, that I am worth a fresh start, that I am worth a man who treats me like an equal? Or, you know, a human being, not just an object or a convenience.

Just letting the women know, just like you came and said we don't deserve it . . . the words, you know, of encouragement and teaching the right way, cuz there's no age limit to learning about your sexuality. And, you know, there's a right way to do things. I'll never be too old to learn how to do the right things. Wisdom comes as you grow old.

Larry: For me, I like to know facts. I like to know why people do things. So I guess trying to figure out what is missing in me that I do these things? Or from like a psychological standpoint, I guess going back to figuring out why I use drugs and why sexuality kind of prompted that.

Casey: So I think helping with self-esteem would help you be more comfortable in what you really want and need sexually.

Linda: What I think is best to me in that area is to . . . go out and sit in groups, and actually just listen and take some suggestions on different strategies that I can take to start learning more about how to better myself and love myself more and care for myself more. Because damage down the line is in my addiction has come about, now that I'm sober, I'm willing to get suggestions on the outside to take in and go along with what I'm willing to do to change my life and start loving myself and caring for myself more.

The honesty and experiences that were shared in the focus groups illustrate how hungry these clients are for information and skills on how to better take care of their sexual health needs and not be further damaged by repeating past behaviors. Promoting positive sexual health through education and activities can help to facilitate this process. We just need the courage to open the door. Once opened, healing can begin. Left closed, shame remains.

RESOURCES

Books

Alman, I. (2001). *Doing it: Real people having really good sex*. Berkeley, CA: Conari Press.

Dockett, L. (2002). *Sex talk: Uncensored exercises for exploring what really turns you on*. Oakland, CA: New Harbinger Publications.

Fulbright, Y. K. (2003). *The hot guide to safer sex*. Alameda, CA: Hunter House.

McCarthy, B. W., & McCarthy, M. E. (2009). *Discovering your couple sexual style*. New York: Routledge.

McCarthy, B. W., & Metz, M. E. (2008). *Men's sexual health: Fitness for satisfying sex*. New York: Routledge.

Online Resources

The Center for Growth, Inc. http://www.sextherapyinphiladelphia.com/index.htm.

Sexuality Information and Education Council of the United States. http://www.siecus.org.

World Association for Sexual Health. http://www.worldsexology.org/millennium-declaration.

TEN

Getting to Know You

There's nothing more intimate in life than simply being understood.
And understanding someone else.

—Brad Meltzer, 2011

It's funny; in this era of e-mail and voice mail and all those things that
even I did not grow up with, a plain old paper letter takes on amazing
intimacy.

—Elizabeth Kostova, 2010

I often hear people talk about being intimate with a partner when they
mean they are being sexual. Going back to language, I believe that many
people, because they have negative connotations of "sex," prefer using
terminology that seems softer to them, in particular, women. The truth
of the matter is that we can be intimate with anyone, and being intimate
has nothing to do with sex per se. As defined in Sexual Beingness, intimacy is about the ability to be close to another human being and have that
closeness returned. Of course, there are different levels of intimacy, as
I may be close to my friends or family in ways that I am not with my
spouse or partner.

Inherent in being intimate is the ability to be vulnerable. If I cannot let
down my defenses and trust my partner, how can I truly be intimate with
them? And so, inherent in being vulnerable with others is the ability to
be able to trust them. Substance abusers very typically have had their trust
shattered on multiple layers, often through traumatic, abusive pasts. For

the addicted person in recovery, learning how to work through the wreck-age of the past and to build trust in a support network or sexual partner can present itself with many challenges. But before we talk about ways to address trust and intimacy issues in treatment, it is necessary to under-stand gender differences in how men and women relate to one another in their worlds. Women's and men's unique experiences and unique percep-tions of those experiences will assist counselors in building a foundation of knowledge for interventions.

FEMINIST AND RELATIONAL THEORY AND WOMEN

Feminist theory considers connectedness to be a cornerstone of the way women relate to their world. This connectedness is viewed as a viable tool for understanding women. An inner sense of connectedness with others is a core construct of women's development (Brown & Gilligan, 1992). Without this sense of connectedness, women may feel adrift. For many women, this sense of being disconnected begins in adolescence and may be related to substance abuse in the teen years. Some research indicates that women with substance abuse issues are less likely to have a well-formed emotional support system (Schilit & Gomberg, 1987).

Related to feminist theory, a framework for understanding women's substance abuse difficulties emphasizes the importance of relationships in women's developmental growth. This framework is based on the "rela-tional model" developed by Miller (1976, 1991). This model implies that women have an intense desire to be in relationships and that the sense of self develops through affiliation, interaction, and engagement with others (Miller, 1991). Recognizing that the self is organized and developed in the context of important relationships (Surrey, 1991), it follows that disconnections (e.g., divorce, violence, and sexual abuse) are the source of psychological problems.

According to the relational model, the primary motivation for women throughout life is to establish a strong sense of connection. Women develop a sense of self-worth when their actions arise from and lead back to connection with others. Healthy, growth-fostering relationships create increased vitality, empowerment, self-knowledge, self-worth, and a desire for more connection. Such relationships are mutual, emphatic, creative, and empowering for all participants (Miller, 1976).

Healthy connections are crucial for women; their psychological prob-lems can be traced to disconnection and violations within relationships: familial, personal, or society at large. When a woman is disconnected from others or involved in abusive relationships, she experiences disempowerment, confusion, and diminished vitality and self-worth—fertile ground for addiction. It is for these reasons that addictions counselors should place women clients in environments in which they can develop connections and experience healthy relationships with providers as well as peers.

Similarly, Gilligan's (1993) theoretical and empirical explorations of female identity and moral development conclude that "identity is formed through the gaining of voices or perspectives, and the self is known through the experience of engagement with different points of view" (p. 153). Both theoretical paradigms describe the female maturation process as a distinct process from males. These differences will impact the addiction and recovery process and should be considered when developing effective treatment strategies.

INDIVIDUATION/SEPARATION THEORY AND MEN

In developmental circles, individuation/separation was postulated to explain the process in which infants were attached to their mothers, literally through the womb, and then separated through birth and development as toddlers, children, and adolescents. As children learn trust and self-sufficiency, they are able to venture out from their mothers to learn how to be individuals, separate from their mother's care, and eventually to be autonomous (Mahler, Pine, & Bergman, 2000). This theory did not take into account gender differences. Nancy Chodorow (1999) theorized that boys are pressured into breaking free of the dependency bond with the mother so that they begin to develop their male identities in accordance with the traditional male role norms of self-reliance and autonomy. Girls, on the other hand, are allowed (and expected) to continue to develop emotional bonds with the mother, fostering reliance on others and dependence.

One of the problems with separation for boys is when self-reliance is forced too early, resulting in psychological trauma and a turning away from attachment to caregivers and from connection. When a boy's father expects a young child to not be a "scaredy cat" in situations where he may be afraid and cry, the child is forced into a role he is not developmentally prepared to handle. For example, a scary movie could cause a young boy to be frightened. If the father (or both parents) expected the boy to "be a man" and not be afraid, the child could experience a loss of attachment when what he really needs is to be comforted and reassured, thus reinforcing trust in his caregivers. As boys mature, this traditional male behavior becomes more prevalent, and any signs of relational (or feminine) traits are often squelched by the father figure (and other boys and men) in efforts to raise the boy to be a man. This premature, forced separation can cause ill effects as boys grow into men. Those maladaptive psychological effects may be due in part to the restrictive norms of men's traditional gender roles as well as when there is angst experienced when there is a failure to achieve masculine role ideals.

GENDER ROLE

Societal norms in terms of gender role, although less restrictive for females, are more restrictive for boys and men. Gender role behavior is socially sanctioned for boys, and they are forced into masculine behaviors that subsequently shape their attitudes toward girls and women. The social construction of this behavior takes the form of several unspoken "rules" that American boys learn to internalize from our culture: to be stoic and not show any weakness by showing pain or displaying grief; to show a propensity toward daring, risk taking, violence, and bravado; to strive to achieve dominance and power over others; and to not show feelings of tenderness, dependence, warmth, and empathy.

GENDER ROLE CONFLICT

"Gender role conflict" is a term that has been used to define the traditional attitudes toward male gender roles that cause men psychological strain, for example, when men experience extreme discomfort and angst from engaging in perceived feminine roles, such as being passive, being helpful or caring, and such. This conflict is thought to be a direct result from maladaptive adjustments from the separation-individuation process. William Pollack (1995) has proposed that the separation-individuation experience involves psychological trauma for boys that is both normative in male development and consequential for adult men's capacities for intimacy and vulnerability to depression. Gender role conflict occurs when rigid, sexist, or restrictive gender roles have a negative impact on self or others and ultimately are responsible for creating men's fear of the feminine (O'Neil, 2006).

The fear of the feminine is a key concept in the gender role conflict paradigm and is thought to be responsible for producing six patterns of role conflict:

1. Restricted emotionality
2. Socialized control
3. Power and competition

4. Homophobia
5. Restricted sexual and affectionate behaviors
6. Obsession with success and achievement

I maintain that the effects of such gender role conflict, coupled with being raised as a male in U.S. culture, only serve to perpetuate social problems, such as domestic violence, depression, sexism, heterosexism, violence against other men, workaholism, hate, and intolerance, to name a few. When we restrict the parameters of how men are allowed or not allowed to express themselves and allow them to put down and degrade women in the process, we effectively create a social climate that inhibits the expression of intimacy in relationships as well.

INTIMACY AND ITS RELEVANCE TO RELATIONSHIPS

As defined by Advocates for Youth (2011), sexual intimacy is the ability to be emotionally close to another human being and to accept closeness in return. Several aspects of intimacy include sharing, caring, liking or loving another person, emotional risk taking, and vulnerability. Sharing intimacy is part of what makes personal relationships meaningful. The ability to show others that we understand and feel their happiness and their pain demonstrates caring. Experiencing the feelings of another can be uncomfortable to us. Intimacy cannot exist without demonstrating to another our feelings and emotions. Having emotional attachment or connection to others is a manifestation of intimacy. To have true intimacy with others, a person must open up and share feelings and personal information. Sharing personal thoughts and feelings with someone else is risky because the other person may not feel the same way. But it is not possible to be really close with another person without being honest and open with them. And finally, in order to be intimate, vulnerability must be reciprocated as well. To have intimacy means that we share and care, like or love, and take emotional risks. That makes us vulnerable—the person with whom we share, about whom we care, and whom we like or love has the power to hurt us emotionally. Intimacy requires vulnerability on the part of each person in the relationship.

The term "skin hunger" refers to our need to be touched, and with addiction, intimacy can take the form of sexual relationships in order to get one's skin hunger needs met. Young people are not touched as frequently by parents as infants and toddlers are, so in order to get those needs met, young people often look to their peers for touch needs. Sometimes this behavior turns sexual when the real need stems from lack of physical touch:

> I wasn't promiscuous, but I had, there were certain periods in my life where I had lots of sex, and it was with people that I knew, it wasn't with strangers or anything. But there was a period where I had a lot of sex when I drank a lot. And with regard to vulnerability, I had that, and risk taking and skin hunger, you know, just wanting to be touched, and I had problems with that, and that's what I wanted, I wanted someone to like me, I wanted someone to like me, love me, and I would pick people that were wrong for me. I think that it was because of low self-esteem, let me take this person because no one else is going to want me, so let me take the first thing that comes along.

CONNECTIONS TO SUBSTANCE USE

For women, enmeshment and overdependence early on with the primary caregiver relationship can affect the healthy separation process, resulting in what has colloquially been referred to in recovery language as "codependency." Women's involvement with subsequent relationships may be fraught with feelings and behaviors that defer to male power and leave her vulnerable to the wishes and desires of romantic partners. Many women are introduced to substances through a romantic partner, and connections between substance use and relationships may become intertwined. A society that perpetuates unrealistic ideals and models of what romantic relationships look like does a terrible disservice to girls and women when they expect to be romanced, swept off their feet, and cared for by a man. These beliefs can be internalized and result in girls and women giving their power away to a relationship in order to feel good about themselves. And when those relationships involve drugs and alcohol, similar behavioral patterns may emerge.

Client Experiences

Casey: I lost my virginity when I was 14, and when I first go into relationships I was, like, if my boyfriend wasn't affectionate towards me or didn't want to hold my hand, I felt, like, neglected. I didn't know, I was never really taught, I just kind of felt neglected, I had abandonment issues. So when I started dating, it was to fill something that I was lacking somewhere, some love that I felt like I wasn't receiving, so therefore I wanted to constantly feel love or affection from someone. In the risk-taking thing, if they wasn't putting in as much as I was putting in, I felt like the same thing, neglect or abandonment.

Linda: I want to be touched, it's like an attention thing for me, and that's how I learned to get attention was in a sexual way. Even when I was being molested as a child, I remember going back to that situation because I liked the attention, cuz I wasn't getting it at home I guess.

DRUGS AND ALCOHOL AS INTIMATE PARTNER

Drugs and alcohol are psychoactive, meaning that they alter a person's perceptions, feelings, and realities. They also serve to alter consciousness and initially have pleasant side effects; otherwise, why would people bother to use them? Similar to relationships with people, women can develop relationships with their substances if those substances consistently provide positive rewards, take away emotional pain, and serve as surrogate partners:

Andrea: I eventually started using alcohol so I could feel vulnerable so that I could be intimate with other people without putting on the brakes in my own head cuz alcohol releases the inhibitions, so to love me to be a part of and of course eventually made me because my friends were alcoholics, they didn't drink the way that I did. And eventually it led to loss of intimacy, and the only way I could feel intimate or vulnerable was with my best friend [alcohol].

Mandy: My way of getting people to like me was to buy their affection, or buy their love, buy their friendship. And I would push myself on people to try to get them to like me because I never felt a part of, I never felt like I fit in. So that's probably where my biggest circle [of sexuality] connection would be is that I had absolutely no self-esteem. I was capable of loving other people, but I wasn't capable of loving myself. So I needed that outer attention in order to feel somewhat full, and I wasn't still getting it, so I turned to drugs.

For men, intimacy experiences can be minimal. Often, sexual activity equates to intimacy with another person. Messages boys and men receive have to do with achieving status and power, and that can take the form of sexual prowess with women:

Larry: Once I hit high school and I grew up a little bit and lost the weight, became out over the edge of being awkward I had many girlfriends and I had lots of sex so—I don't know. I didn't do it

to be cool. I just did it because that's what we did. I had a steady
girlfriend that I stayed with from sophomore year until senior
year, but there was that time when you break off and then go
with someone else and then come back, and that usually
involved sex. So I had multiple, multiple partners for years.

Over time, as men mature and develop a sense of identity that involves
more of themselves as individuals, the meaning of the "conquest" can lose
its meaning if the loneliness of addiction and meaningless sexual activity
are the impetus for change. The place of intimacy can shift with development and the recovery process:

Barry: As I got older, though, I could really understand what skin
hunger was and things like that. After we separated, I went
overseas, so the last time there was a span of several years
before I had sex again, and during that time I continued to abuse
my body, and I would drink. And so my whole identity was I
was never going to be intimate with anybody. I was never going
to be able to because I'm a wreck, I'm a drunk, I'm ruined, and
this continued through my thirties. I basically shot the whole
decade in my thirties, my prime. I continued to do really well in
work, move up that way, and they love an alcoholic that's
functional, so I was able to do that well. I was traveling all the
time, but I was never attracted—attractable—or no one found
me attractive even in my mind, and I continued to lose any kind
of sexual personality. And it wasn't until I hooked up with an
old girlfriend from my childhood that I had sex again, and it felt
really cool, and that lasted for a couple times, and then it went
away until I met my second wife, and then it was very good,
very, very good, and I was sober. And that's when I really loved
the intimacy and the feeling and the touching and I realized
what a healthy body image was like. I realized what being
touched was like and all that.

Being able to help clients make the connections between their past relationships, learned intimacy patterns, and connections to substance use is a
critical step in facilitating a sense of what healthy relationships look like,
both sexual and nonsexual. The following ideas for activities can be useful
in helping clients to explore how the past connects to the present in terms
of how they relate to others and their abilities to recognize and define positive qualities in a relationship.

IDEAS FOR GROUP ACTIVITIES TO EXPLORE INTIMACY AND RELATIONSHIPS

We do not exist in a vacuum. Most of us have friends and family with whom we cultivate close relationships. Whether it consists of a day out with the gals shopping or a night on the town or playing horseshoes or playing ball with the guys, we all have the need for closeness to other human beings. We find meaning in life through our connections to others. Depending on our past experiences with friends and family, we all develop individual patterns of behavior and reactions based on those initial experiences. If our past friendships were fraught with stress, abuse, and mistrust, we may have more difficulty in making connections in adulthood. Examining our past can give us direction to make positive changes with regard to unhealthy relationship patterns.

It can be helpful for people in treatment to begin to examine their relationships with friends and family in order to identify any dysfunctional patterns. If we are male and Dad was cold, distant, and disapproving, we may not have learned how to be close with our male friends or our sons. An interesting activity that has been used in psychotherapy and can be helpful in treatment is called the family sculpture. A psychological underpinning of this activity is known as corrective emotional recapitulation (Yalom, 1970). Corrective emotional recapitulation occurs when we reexperience an emotional event from our past in order to work through emotions that might still keep us stuck emotionally. This commonly happens with substance abusers. There are a number of ways this type of activity can be facilitated; I will describe two ways I have used it in treatment groups.

THE FICTITIOUS FAMILY SCULPTURE

In the event you do not have an identified client issue to work with or decide that it would be less threatening to use an activity that is fictitious, another way to facilitate the activity is to create a fictitious scenario that has several parts: preevent, event, postevent. For example, you can create a fictitious family using group members (with the same number of group members in the present group): father, mother, siblings, and maybe an aunt or uncle or two if necessary. Alternatively, ask one or two members to be observers. All the assigned group members get ages and birth placement so that they know how they are all related. In the first scenario, let them interact with each other as a normal family for about 5 to 10 minutes.

The group then receives news that the mother just found out she has cancer; the counselor does not have to provide details of the cancer, the mother can decide what kind of cancer she has, and so on. So, her tasks in the next role play might include issues of disclosure and who and how to tell about it. Allow at least 10 minutes for the second part of the role play so that the family members can interact with one another.

In the third scenario, the mother has progressed, a year has passed, and all treatments have failed; her death will be imminent. Again, let the group role-play for another 10 minutes.

In the final scenario, after a few more months, the mother has died. The group should role-play for the last 10 minutes about how they continue to deal with the death and their relationships with each other.

The counselor should have the scenarios memorized ahead or be able to read them off a sheet to the group as the activity progresses and should be cognizant of group dynamics and how the "family" relationships play out. Observers can either take notes or make mental observations to process the activity when it is complete. Typically, with this activity, family-of-origin issues surface and group members take on specific roles they had from their own families of origin. The role plays can get quite heated and emotional. Some process questions for after the group is complete include the following:

1. What was this activity like for you? Allow only one person to share at a time.
2. What was it like to find out about the initial diagnosis?
3. How did you feel when you found out that your mother (or you, the mother figure) was dying?
4. After the mother died, what was going on for you? How did you cope with the loss?
5. What observations do you have about yourself with regard to your reactions and your relationships with the family as the activity progressed?
6. What patterns did anyone notice about how your reactions from this activity relate to your real life and/or connections to your substance use?

When I process family sculpture activities, I typically do them with myself as part of the group in a circle in order to be present with emotional reactions. Once the process is complete, I always ask the group members to shake off their family role—ask them to get up and say out loud that "I am not the big sister, mother, and so on." This symbolically allows them to disconnect with any negative associations of their roles.

If there is time in the session, a brief brainstorming activity should be conducted. Using a whiteboard or blank newsprint taped to a wall, write the words "positive" and "not so positive." Ask the group to come up with characteristics regarding their communication styles that fit under both categories; these can include verbal and nonverbal traits. Completing the group in this manner also allows for participants to debrief in a less emotional manner and includes another learning style: visual.

Whichever of these activities is used, they can be a good lead-in for a second activity the following week, that is, to examine what personality traits improve or damage relationships and how one feels about relationships. The use of journaling can be a powerful homework assignment between groups.

ACTIVITY: INTIMACY IN RELATIONSHIPS

In preparation for the second session on intimacy and relationships, four pieces of newsprint should be prepared with the following written at the top of each sheet: (1) family members (siblings parents grandparents, aunts, uncles, and so on), (2) friends, (3) professional relationships (bosses, business associates, colleagues, counselors, and legal and social workers), and (4) romantic partners. The group should be divided so that two or three people each have one of the topics. Each group's task is to brainstorm what characteristics enhance these relationships and which traits can damage them. The sheets should be divided side by side or top/bottom. Give each group about 15 minutes to complete the task.

Facilitate a discussion of their process and feelings using the following questions:

1. How did it feel to do this?
2. What do you notice about the positive things listed for the different relationships?
3. What do you notice about the negative things?
4. Were any parts difficult to do? Why or why not?
5. Were there any similarities in positives or negatives among the sheets? If so, what were they?
6. How might internalizing these messages be harmful as we try to stay clean and sober?

Discussion Points

To follow this up in group, conduct a brainstorming activity in which group members define which components they feel are integral to healthy relationships. Ask for ideas and record them on newsprint (or a white-board). Once all the components are identified, process with the following discussion questions:

1. If you had to give up one quality in your relationship with someone important in your life, which would you be most willing to give up? What about in a relationship with a friend? Romantic partner? Why?
2. Which of the qualities would you be unwilling to ever give up? Why?
3. How would you feel about someone who did not respect you? Who did not put enough work into the relationship? What could you do about it?
4. Which qualities do you think are the most difficult to find in a relationship?
5. How does this affect the relationships you currently have in your life?
6. How might it affect your ability to stay clean and sober?

NEXT STEPS

Society often upholds the idea that intimacy is just about sexual relationships when intimacy is about the ability to be close to another human being and have that closeness returned. This includes a variety of relationships, nonsexual as well as sexual. Many substance-abusing persons have learned unhealthy sexual practices that mimic intimacy through sex and can benefit from learning perspectives to view intimacy in a broader context. Teaching clients how to identify how intimacy has played itself out in the context of family-of-origin relationships can help them to connect these patterns of relating to their current situations and connections to their subsequent substance use. Making these connections will help counselors to address relapse prevention and find ways to enhance the recovery process for clients.

RESOURCES

Books

Carlson, J., & Sperry, L. (2010). *Recovering intimacy in love relationships: A clinician's guide.* New York: Routledge.
Karen, R. (1998). *Becoming attached.* New York: Oxford University Press.
Kasl, C. (1997). *A home for the heart: A practical guide to intimate and social relationships.* New York: HarperCollins.

Keesling, B. (2005). *Sexual pleasure: Reaching new heights of sexual arousal and intimacy.* Alameda, CA: Hunter House.

Metz, M. E., & McCarthy, B. W. (2011). *Enduring desire: Your guide to lifelong intimacy.* New York: Taylor & Francis.

Prager, K. (1995). *The psychology of intimacy.* New York: Guilford Press.

Robins, S. P. (2010). *Exploring intimacy: Cultivating healthy relationships through insight and intuition.* New York: Rowman & Littlefield.

Online Resources

Building Intimacy. http://sexualintimacyboulder.com.

Family Resource. http://www.familyresource.com/relationships/building-and-maintaining/the-impact-of-intimacy.

The Intimate Couple. http://www.the-intimate-couple.com/intimacy-problems.html.

ELEVEN

Oh God!

What we do comes out of who we believe we are.

—Rob Bell

Spirituality. Religion. God. What images came to your mind when you read these three words? Many of us have strong reactions when we are faced with our feelings of faith, both positive and negative, depending on our experiences over the life span. Spirituality is related to a person's internal moral compass, feelings of connection to a power greater than ourselves, a heart connection to life and beyond. For many individuals, this spirituality is "housed" under the formal framework of a religion or practice. But for others, it may lie within them as an ethical framework in which to operate in the world. Either way, spirituality and sexual health should include alignment between one's ethical, spiritual, and moral beliefs and one's sexual behaviors and values. Based on the lived experiences of people with substance use problems, there are often discrepancies between the two.

RELIGIOSITY AND SPIRITUALITY, THE GLUE THAT HOLDS IT ALL TOGETHER

There are differences between religiosity and spirituality, although some people use the terms interchangeably. Religiosity and spirituality can be defined broadly as any feelings, thoughts, experiences, and behaviors that arise from a search for the "sacred," with the former implying group or social practices and doctrines and the latter tending to refer to personal experiences and beliefs (Hill et al., 2000). Religiousness/religiosity can also be viewed as a set of behaviors (social or private, including rituals), values, and attitudes that are based on (and that lie within the boundaries of) previously established religious doctrine and institutionalized organization; spirituality can be viewed as an unbounded set of personal drives, behaviors, experiences, values, and attitudes that are related to existential understanding, meaning, purpose, and transcendence. Although one does not preclude the other, people who do not identify with an organized religion have the propensity to have spiritual connections in life.

Spirituality seems to involve connection and the interconnectedness of all things in life: people, nature, and a higher purpose. It is this interconnectedness that leads people to seek the good in others, suggesting an altruistic (social justice and love for humanity) component. A healthy spirituality, then, is not a matter of living in isolation but of living in harmony with other people. Human beings seek meaning and purpose in life (Wulff, 1991). With addiction, if people do not find meaning in life, existential angst is created, resulting in an emotional void. Some people attempt to fill the void with things such as sex, drugs, or alcohol—a search for meaning outside of self. And in recovery circles, particularly Narcotics Anonymous, the statement "one is too many, a thousand never enough" refers to those attempts to fill the void with substances.

People want to understand the universe, the nature of humanity and the relationship to all things in life. Faith provides us with the motivation to confront our problems. Our spirituality develops when we put it into action. Action happens through prayer or meditation and allows us to listen to the inner voice—this is what we call the life force or God—and it gives us direction. Helping the recovering person to reconnect to this force can be a powerful and positive influence.

MORALITY, SUBSTANCE USE, AND SEXUALITY

There are similarities between a morality that views sexual activities outside a prescribed relationship (e.g., between a married man and his wife) as deviant and the consumption of alcohol and other drugs. In the field of addiction, this is known as the moral model. The moral model frames addiction as a result of human weakness, a defect in character. It doesn't recognize biological or genetic components to addiction and offers little sympathy for those who display addictive behaviors. The implication is that addiction is the result of poor choices that addicts make because of a lack of willpower or moral strength. Treatment outcomes associated with the moral model include disdain for substance abusers, low tolerance for relapse and harm reduction approaches, judgmental approaches, and so on. This approach is not conducive to recovery.

HISTORICAL VIEWS OF ADDICTION

Unsurprisingly, viewing addiction as a moral failing led alcoholics and other addicts to be grouped with others who had demonstrated "moral failings," such as the mentally ill and criminals. In the nineteenth and early twentieth centuries, alcoholism was associated with other socially undesirable situations and behaviors, such as crime, poverty, sin, domestic violence, and laziness. Rather than proposing treatment methods for alcoholism, the moral model viewed punishment as a more appropriate response. Alcoholics were reluctant to publicly acknowledge their problem, as society had little sympathy for their struggle. So, of course, these people were to blame if they suffered other consequences, such as sexual assault, rape, sexual dysfunctions, and so on. Didn't they just "ask for it" when they were under the influence? The resulting belief that they also "deserved" what happened to them is still transparent today. A perfect example of this is when individuals comment on people with HIV who became infected through sexual behaviors and state that they "deserve what they got" (as a result of their sinful behaviors, such as perceived sexual permissiveness and/or homosexual activity).

IMPACT OF HISTORY

Although this model does not dominate the treatment field today, its roots shaped public attitude toward substance use; the effects are seen in the criminal justice system, for example. Rather than receiving treatment, many individuals are still incarcerated for substance-related infractions of the law. The idea that a person can "pull themselves up by the bootstraps" reinforces the belief that overcoming addiction is about willpower, and this in turn reinforces the moral model: if you were not weak in character, you could overcome this problem. Call it blaming the victim.

Some of the resulting emotional damage from a person internalizing these views can be exacerbated by accompanying sexual behaviors that are similarly viewed as "deviant" or unacceptable forms of expression. Going back to the roots of a moralistic view of sexuality, we can make connections between the multiple stigmas of substance use and aspects of sexual behaviors. The more layered the stigma, the greater the resulting feelings of shame. It is almost impossible to live in a culture that views sex and substance use as a moral deficiency and not internalize the beliefs at some level. Repeatedly hearing these values affects us all to some degree.

LEARNED MESSAGES

Finding solace and meaningful connections to our spirit often take on more relevance through the life span, and many folks who turn to substances for comfort have unresolved issues related to their spirit. Over my years of work in the field, clients have consistently reported this unresolved or ambivalent relationship with their god or their moral compass. Many of them were raised with shaming messages about different aspects of their sexuality, and direct connections were noted in many of our interviews:

Linda: My mother is a minister, and so is my stepfather. So I was brought up, I guess you could say, traditional, really didn't talk about sex. But when we did, I was taught that girls and boys are supposed to be together, if not you'll burn in hell, and basically that's it. No homosexuality, none of that stuff, it was looked down upon. Basically you'll go to hell.

Mandy: What I learned about sexuality was that it stayed quiet. Nobody is to know about what you do. And that's not from the parents, it's from the cousins. And at church it's like, you don't have sex period, you're gonna burn. So it's like whatever you do, don't let the grown-ups know. So that's what I learned about sex.

Learning how to hide sexuality contributes to feelings of guilt and shame. When we have to hide aspects of ourselves, the driving messages tell us that those aspects are wrong and that we should be ashamed of them. Unfortunately, some of these messages are derived from religious beliefs. But the Bible does not say that sex is a sin; what becomes twisted is the interpretation of those messages and how they are conveyed. When we go back to the idea that religion was used as a way to control people's behaviors, it makes sense that the perceived undesirable behaviors are the ones that are condemned. And when a larger part of a community shuns individuals for engaging in behaviors, the power of shame becomes an intense force:

Andrea: I was firmly raised as a Lutheran, and I always wanted to wait till I was married, and I still wish I could've waited till I was married. And that's what my parents taught me, and I really believe that that's what's right, but once it's gone its gone, and there's nothing you can do about it.

Barry: And then with the sex, I always felt like I was doing something dirty, so I would drink, and that was when I just felt like I was doing something wrong. The more I drank and did whatever I was doing, then I could do it if I needed to or whatever, but I always felt like it was something wrong, and I was raised Catholic as well, so I think that had a lot to do with it.

Of course, not all stories were fraught with such dichotomies. And those were far and few between, but one person had shared the following:

Larry: I guess when I, my impressionable years when I really took it in at a Catholic school, sex was talked about in the procreation manner and between a husband and a wife. There were the older kids that would take pledges not to engage in sex, and there were certain things like that, but there was never really a sex education; there was more like a health class. There really wasn't what the public schools had. I don't think but the messages I got was that sex was good.

The message that sex was good is absent from the schema of most of the clients we interviewed. The underlying message they shared was that their behaviors went against what was acceptable and good. And even for the person who shared that the messages about sex were good struggled to have a healthy sexuality because of his addiction and a poor self-image.

Guilt and shame associated with sexual activities that are not congruent with an addicted person's self-defined morals and standards can lead to the use of substances in order to lessen these feelings. Feeling guilt and shame about sexual activities (masturbation, sex outside of marriage, same-sex behaviors, divorce, abortion, multiple partners) have been directly linked to religious values and can cause a great deal of personal angst for clients as they explore sexual behaviors that may go against their religious upbringing. Internalizing this shame can be problematic for a number of reasons, including damage resulting from self-blame over sexual abuse and nonconsensual sexual events as well as sexual revictimization (Braun-Harvey, 2009; Runtz, 2003; Shapiro & Schwarz, 1997).

FINDING MEANING

Using substances can be an attempt for people to connect to something outside of them and to find meaning in life, but the compulsive use of substances can also lead to feelings of emptiness and a void unfulfilled. When people use substances to mask sexual feelings or engage in sexual behavior, disconnection from the spirit occurs. Helping someone to find congruence between one's ethical, spiritual and moral beliefs, and sexual behaviors and values is an important component of sexual health. And this connection need not be tied only to formal religion but may also include ethical and moral concerns. All of our clients should be encouraged to reflect on their deeper values to find ways to integrate their sexual and spiritual selves in the expectation that this will lead to a more successful recovery trajectory.

Connecting to the Process

What can we do to foster this reconnection to spirit? Again, it will depend on the individual's personal values and beliefs, but working with people to have them learn what they *do* believe is part of the solution. As was mentioned earlier, the use of values clarification activities in a sexual health group can facilitate this personal growth to promote healing. Looking at values in sexual health is critical in order to help participants consider how their values impact certain behaviors. If sexuality education is taught from one viewpoint, without challenging learners to examine their beliefs and have the opportunity to obtain information from multiple views, the options and abilities of individuals to make informed or healthy choices that make sense to them will be limited. If controversial subjects are taught, then a range of viewpoints must be discussed and reviewed in the context of a rational, democratic philosophy (Gilgun & Gordon, 1983). Information and group discussion will involve participants in discussing a variety of views and options.

A sexuality and addiction timeline can help clients to ascertain the links between any sexual and substance linked behaviors. Helping clients to make these connections can enable them to develop a treatment plan that addresses how relapse is inextricably related to certain sexual connections. And in doing so, not only can clients learn to lessen any sexual shame; they can learn healthy ways to be sexual and satisfied in relationships. Talking about sex and planning for future situations reduces the risk for relapse.

By asking clients to look at how they feel about their substance use, their sexual behaviors associated with substance use, and their connection to their spirituality, a sense of ownership occurs. Many individuals lose their spiritual connectedness through the misuse of substances, so getting clean and sober is a starting point. Twelve-step facilitation can help some people reconnect to a "god of their understanding." For others, inner reflection through the use of values clarification, group process and discussion, sentence completion homework, and journaling are excellent tools for helping them connect to a sense of their spirit.

Spiritual journeys are another venue that creates a space for personal exploration such as meditation, vision quests, drumming circles, holistic workshops, and so on. One recovering woman I worked with had reconnected to her spirit after a divorce by going on a woman's backpacking journey in the Pecos Wilderness of New Mexico, a deeply spiritual place. During her journey, she made profound personal discoveries through the group work and took on a spirit name from her vision quest experience. The renaming helped her to separate from the sexual abuse she had experienced and take back her personal power over sexual shame. This was several years into her recovery, illustrating that dealing with past sexual abuse is a process. More importantly it was a process she was aware of because we had worked with her sexuality and addiction linked shame.

These reconnections take time and patience. Is the loss of a spiritual center an issue that your clients bring to the table? We must take care not to force our values or beliefs on clients in terms of spirituality and sexuality. We need to be able to guide individuals toward what makes sense to them in their lives, with their families, and with their peer groups. Those clients who are at odds with a religious affiliation may need alternatives to 12-step facilitation, such as rational recovery or women for sobriety or other wellness options. Not pushing them into a box where they don't fit is critical to building trust in the therapeutic relationship; having alternatives to 12-step meetings for support will be helpful for working with clients who reject traditional religious ideas. And for those who became disconnected from their religious upbringing because of substance use and its outcomes, helping them reconnect to their spirit will be integral to the recovery process.

RESOURCES

Books

Bien, T., & Bien, B. (2002). *Mindful recovery: A spiritual path to healing from addiction*. New York: John Wiley.

Gregson, D., & Efran, J. S. (2002). *The Tao of sobriety: Helping you to recover from alcohol and drug addiction*. New York: St. Martin's Press.

Shapiro, R. (2009). *Recovery—The sacred art: The twelve steps as spiritual practice*. Woodstock, VT: SkyLight Paths.

Tigert, L. M., & Brow, T. (2001). *Coming out young and faithful*. Cleveland, OH: Pilgrim Press.

TWELVE

Completing the Journey

Only one who, tragically, has never experienced love would question whether sex can be fulfilling when love is absent. Physically satisfying, perhaps, but never fulfilling. It can never reach the depths of what we are as human beings, and what we are capable of becoming. To climb the heights, sex education is not enough.
We need to learn how to love.

—Joseph and Lois Bird, 1976

As we complete our journey around Sexual Beingness, my hope is that you are coming away with a deeper understanding of the complexities involved with incorporating sexual health programming into the treatment realm. Sexuality is multifaceted, and each area can have a profound effect on the recovery trajectories of those who are impacted by substance use. Having the ability to develop sensitivity to and knowledge of how sexuality affects the addiction and recovery process will increase the likelihood of successful outcomes.

A holistic approach to recovery incorporates a myriad of techniques that include sexual health. Conceptualizing sexual health broadly is holistic. We are all sexual beings and cannot separate our sexual selves from our emotions and beliefs. Recovery is about change, and in order to facilitate healthy change, we must consider all those things that contributed to the problematic use of substances, including the sexual self.

SEXUAL HEALTH AND ADDICTION TREATMENT MODEL

Sexuality has been ignored too long in the treatment realm. A theoretical framework for addressing sexuality in treatment utilizes a model that I have developed with my colleague and foreword writer Douglas Braun-Harvey; I call this the Sexual Health Addiction Treatment Model (Figure 12.1). It begins with sexuality issues linked to the use of substances. The resulting data in the research model is directly linked to intimacy, sexualization, shame, sexual health and reproduction, sexual identity and sensuality. In order to treat these connected sexual variables, a sexual health intervention must be provided. Prior studies showed improved treatment outcomes and client retention as a result of sexual health programming (Braun-Harvey, 2009 & 2010).

Interrupting the internal process and negative self-dialogue are things that I believe need to be addressed for clients in treatment programs in order for them to successfully recover, stay in treatment and help prevent relapse. Many relapse triggers for substance-using clients include latent, unresolved sexual issues. Addressing sexuality in treatment programs may provide a baseline for new understanding and help counselors to set up a vital follow-up treatment plan that includes awareness and understanding of sexuality issues that may need further therapy, support, and intervention.

By providing this vital information and experience to chemically dependent clients, we can begin to break a model of "labeling," misdiagnosing, and maltreating. Instead of perpetuating a model that promotes powerlessness and internal shame over feeling defective or deviant, we can offer hope of sexual healing and give a unique opportunity for recovering people to feel good about who they are and empower them to reclaim their sexuality as special, precious, and healthy for them.

Shifting the emphasis from the negative to the positive, giving people power over their destinies, and allowing for self-actualization is the mainstay of treatment from addiction. Sexual health groups can provide positive role modeling and help clients to normalize sexual feelings, develop interpersonal skills, and build support networks and, through shared experiences, help them recognize societal patterns of sexual oppression. Creating an emotionally safe and supportive environment allows clients in treatment to address issues of sexual, physical, and emotional abuse at a rate and intensity appropriate for each individual.

Assessing clients for low sexual self-esteem is one way to identify specific variables for treatment planning and also to use as a marker for improvement over time. Increased scores of sexual self-esteem measured

Figure 12.1   Hypothesized Model of Sexuality and Addiction.

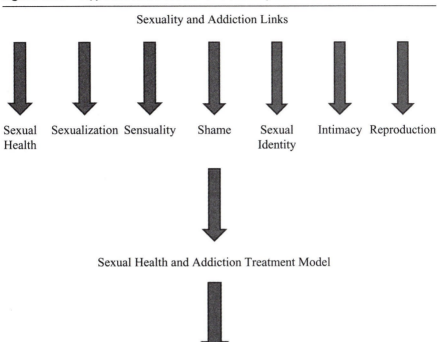

Sexuality and Addiction Links

Sexual   Sexualization Sensuality   Shame   Sexual   Intimacy Reproduction
Health   Identity

Sexual Health and Addiction Treatment Model

Improved Treatment Outcomes/Client Retention

over time will inform clinicians of progress during and after treatment. Continued aftercare and support services can help providers to track sexuality-related relapse related to a number of sexual health issues.

THOUGHTS ON DEVELOPING EFFECTIVE INTERVENTIONS

The National Institutes of Health has several branches that deal specifically with substance abuse prevention, treatment, and research. The National Institute on Drug Abuse developed a mechanism in the 1990s that specifies a systematic process for developing behavioral interventions. Substance abuse is linked to environmental, genetic, cultural, biological, and behavioral causes; therefore, treatment for substance use disorders includes many different approaches, including pharmacological, psychological, and behavioral methods. Initially, treatment for substance use disorders consisted of 12-step facilitation based in part on the disease model, and many counselors at the time were also recovering from substance use disorders. As other models of addiction were developed and became integrated, approaches for treatment slowly began to change. Newer treatments and approaches, including motivational interviewing, cognitive-behavioral therapy, harm reduction, and new drugs, such as Suboxone for opiate addiction, are quite efficacious in working with specific types of clients at differing levels of recovery over time. Within the field of addiction, varying beliefs and approaches that can be employed can make it difficult for program staff to agree on how to best treat their clients. The addictions field is one of the only counseling specialties that does not have a systematic framework for educational requirements and training of counselors, although with managed care, requirements for credentialed addiction counselors are being raised in many states to the master's level. I feel that as an individual seeking treatment, I would want the person treating me to be educated in all techniques and approaches in order to employ a comprehensive, individualized assessment and treatment plan. And just as we are all unique with our life experiences, a one-size-fits-all approach will not work with every client. Being able to incorporate an eclectic approach that encourages counselors to individually assess and choose methods that match the individual is recommended.

The behavioral therapies development program of the National Institute on Drug Abuse allows for new treatments to be developed, piloted for efficacy, and tested scientifically if its outcomes are shown to be promising. Along with developing behavioral interventions, manuals are written and counselors are trained in how to effectively implement treatment; these are alternatively referred to as empirically supported treatments or manualized treatment. One problem with manualized treatment is that many counselors feel that the manuals are too scripted and employ a cookie-cutter approach, taking the individuality of counselor skill and abilities out of the equation. Another issue I have observed is that once counselors are trained in a particular method, they often do not stick to the manual 100 percent of the time. In research, these are limitations of human factors that can impact the efficacy of programming outcomes. Other research has demonstrated that it does not necessarily matter which type of treatment is used but that counselor attributes account for a large percentage of positive client outcomes.

The point I am trying to make is about making treatment manuals flexible, giving counselors a choice of materials, and allowing them to be able to individually assess a particular group of clients and then choosing the activities or lessons that can best address the issues that are being presented rather than imposing a rigid curricula that may not be the best fit. I am currently conducting research that falls under behavioral therapies development and proposing a sexual health curriculum that truly lives up to a stage model of change. My current project focuses on women's sexual health; the curriculum is being developed for pilot testing as I write this book. I hope to help revolutionize approaches for the use of manualized treatment in the addictions field. In the meantime, I give ideas to you on how to conceptualize the links between sexuality and addiction. I also give to you ideas for incorporating sexual health programming into the work you currently are doing with clients. Finally, I hope you take this information to heart; it may just save someone's life.

APPENDIX A

Sexual History Intake Questions Sensitive to Sexual Diversity

Listed below are several questions that may be used during the initial interview. Some of these questions will be appropriate for your services while others may not. Adopt the questions to meet your personal needs, needs of the client, and the needs of your organization/agency. Respecting where the client is with regard to their sexuality is of utmost importance.

Legal name:

Preferred name (if different):

Sex/Gender:
❑ Male
❑ Female
❑ Transgender
❑ Male to female
❑ Female to male
❑ Other (Describe): _____

Are your current sexual partners men? women? or both?

In the past, have your sexual partners been men? women? or both?

How do you describe your sexual identity?
❑ Straight/heterosexual
❑ Lesbian

❑ Gay
❑ Bisexual
❑ Queer
❑ Other (Describe): _____
❑ Questioning
❑ Don't know

What is your current relationship status?
❑ Single
❑ Marriage to opposite sex
❑ Same-sex marriage/common law
❑ Partnered
❑ Involved with multiple partners
❑ Separated from spouse/partner
❑ Divorced/permanently separated from spouse/partner
❑ Other (Describe):_____

What is your living situation?
❑ Live alone
❑ Live with spouse or partner
❑ Live with roommate(s)
❑ Live with parents or other family members
❑ Other (Describe): _____

Are there any children in your home?
❑ No children in home
❑ My own children live with me/us
❑ My spouse or partner's children live with me/us
❑ Shared custody with ex-spouse/partner

Do you need any information about safer-sex techniques?
If yes, with:
❑ Men
❑ Women
❑ Both

Are you currently experiencing any sexual concerns?

What safer-sex methods or contraceptive methods do you use, if any?

Do you want to start a family?

Are there any questions you have, or information you would like, with respect to starting a family?

Have you or your partner experienced an unplanned pregnancy? If yes, how did you handle it?

Do you have any concerns related to your gender identity?

Do you currently use or have you used hormones? (e.g., estrogen, testosterone, etc.)

Do you need any information on hormone therapy?

Have you ever been tested for HIV?
❑ Yes, most recent test: _____
❑ No
If yes, what was your result_____. When_____ (HIV test results are considered confidential information, regardless of status)

Have you ever been diagnosed with, or treated for, a sexually transmitted infection (STI)?
Yes, I have been tested and/or treated for:
❑ Herpes
❑ Syphilis
❑ Gonorrhea
❑ Chlamydia
❑ HPV/human papilloma virus (causes genital warts & abnormal PAP smears)
❑ HIV/AIDS
❑ Other_____

Would you like more information on STI/HIV?

Would you like more information on how to reduce your risk of getting an STI/HIV?

Have you had any sexual experiences lately that you think may have put you at risk for STI/HIV?

Have you ever used any substances (e.g., alcohol, marijuana, injection drugs) to make you feel good?
If yes, which _____ _____ _____
and when was the last time _____ _____ _____?

Have you come into contact with needles as a result of tattooing, piercing, injection drugs or blood transfusion?
If yes, which _____ _____ _____
and when _____?

Have you ever been diagnosed with, or treated for, hepatitis A, B, and/ or C?
If yes, which and when?

Have you ever been vaccinated against hepatitis A or B?
Vaccinated against hepatitis A
Vaccinated against hepatitis B

Below is a list of risk factors for hepatitis A, B, and C. Do any of these apply to you?
❑ Yes
❑ No
❑ Not sure

Hepatitis Risk Factors (Check all that apply)
Have you ever:
❑ participated in sexual activity that shares blood or fluid
❑ had multiple sex partners
❑ had oral-fecal contact
❑ had sexual activity during a menstrual period
❑ traveled to regions where Hepatitis is common
❑ had a tattoo, or a piercing
❑ used injecting or non-injecting drugs
❑ been diagnosed with or treated for STI/HIV
❑ come into close contact with someone who has Hepatitis A, B or C

APPENDIX B

Sexuality Comfort
Self-Assessment

How Comfortable Are You?
Personal Comfort Self-Assessment
In order to be successful communicating with clients around sexuality issues, staff needs to feel comfortable discussing a variety of topics. This exercise will help you evaluate your own readiness to talk with clients in a variety of relevant topic areas. Please look at each topic and check each box to the right if the statements are true. If the statement is not true, leave a space in that box. In the last column is a space for you to write ideas you have about how to increase your comfort with the topic, such as reading about it, observing others, attending training, asking questions of an experienced staff person, practice talking about it, etc.

Topic	I feel that I have enough knowledge to talk about this topic with a client.	I feel that I have enough experience to talk about this topic with a client.	My own values will not conflict with my ability to talk about this topic with a client.	What I can do to increase my comfort?
Vaginal sex				
Anal sex				
Fellatio (oral sex on a man)				
Cunnilingus (oral sex on a woman)				
Fisting/rimming				
Abstinence				
Masturbation				
Human sexual response cycle				
Sex with multiple partners				
Sex toys (vibrators, dildos)				
Group sex				
Abortion				
Infertility				
Sexual dysfunction				
Birth control				
Alternative methods of reproducing				

Out-of-control sexual
  behaviors
Extrarelational sex
  (cheating)
Fantasy
Sexual abuse
Rape
Swinging
Fetishes
Bondage, dominance,
  sadomasochism
  (BDSM)
Others? Please list

APPENDIX C

Values Clarification

Read each statement and circle the appropriate response.
SA = Strongly Agree, A = Agree, N = Neutral, D = Disagree,
SD = Strongly Disagree

1. Condoms should always be used when a person has sex.

   SA   A   N   D   SD

2. A person should be free to express their sexual orientation.

   SA   A   N   D   SD

3. People with HIV should disclose their status to coworkers and colleagues.

   SA   A   N   D   SD

4. Condoms should always be used when a person with an STI has sex.

   SA   A   N   D   SD

5. Women with HIV should not get pregnant or have babies.

   SA   A   N   D   SD

6. Bisexuals are to blame for the spread of HIV to heterosexuals.

   SA   A   N   D   SD

7. Injection drug users deserve to get infected.

   SA   A   N   D   SD

8. If my sexual partner found out they had an STI, I would end the relationship.

SA   A   N   D   SD

9. Doctors and health care providers have the right to know their patients HIV status.

SA   A   N   D   SD

10. If a pregnant woman finds out she is HIV+, she should terminate the pregnancy.

SA   A   N   D   SD

11. People with HIV/STIs deserve what they get.

SA   A   N   D   SD

12. People with HIV should not have sexual relations.

SA   A   N   D   SD

13. Providing clean needles to drug users is wrong.

SA   A   N   D   SD

Sources

PREFACE

Centers for Disease Control and Prevention. (2009). *HIV surveillance report*. Retrieved September 1, 2011, from http://www.cdc.gov/hiv/surveillance/resources/reports/2009report/pdf/table20.pdf.

National Institute for Drug Abuse. (2011). *Principle of drug addiction treatment: A research-based guide*. Retrieved September 1, 2011, from http://www.nida.nih.gov/podat/faqs.html.

CHAPTER 1

Advocates for Youth. (2011). The circles of human sexuality. Retrieved September 1, 2011, from http://www.advocatesforyouth.org/for-professionals/lesson-plans-professionals/198?task=view.

Bartholomew, K., & Horowitz, L. (1991). Attachment styles of young adults: A test of a four-category model. *Journal of Personality and Social Psychology, 61*(2), 226–44.

Braun-Harvey, D. (2009). *Sexual health in drug and alcohol treatment: A group facilitators manual*. New York: Springer.

Buss, D. M. (1994). *The evolution of desire: Strategies of human mating*. New York: Basic Books.

Daniluk, J. C. (1993). The meaning and experience of female sexuality: A phenomenological analysis. *Psychology of Women Quarterly, 17*, 53–69.

Feeney, J., & Noller, P. (1996). *Adult attachment*. Thousand Oaks, CA: Sage.

Feingold, A. (1992). Good-looking people are not what we think. *Psychological Bulletin, 111*, 304–41.

Fredrickson, B. L., & Roberts, T. (1997). Objectification theory: Toward understanding women's lived experiences and mental health risks. *Psychology of Women Quarterly, 21*, 173–206.

Gaynor, P., & Underwood, J. (1995). Conceptualizing and measuring sexual self-esteem. In S. Shrout & S. Fiske (Eds.), *Personality research, methods and theory: A Festschrift honoring Donald W. Fiske*. Hillsdale, NJ: Lawrence Erlbaum Associates.

Halstead, L. S., & Halstead, K. (1983). Disability SARs and the small group experience: A conceptual framework. *Sexuality and Disability, 6*, 183–96.

Held, J. P., Cournoyer, C. R., Held, C. A., & Chilgren, R. A. (1974). Sexual attitude reassessment: A training seminar for health professionals. *Minnesota Medicine, 57*, 925–28.

James, R. (2011). Correlates of sexual self-esteem in a sample of substance abusing women. *Journal of Psychoactive Drugs, 43*(3), 220–28.

Kirby, D. (2000). What does the research say about sexuality education? *Educational Leadership,* October, 2000, 72–76.

La Cursia, N., Beyer, C., & Ogletree, R. (1994). The importance of a philosophy in sexuality education. *Family Life Educator 13*(1), 4–9.

Lawrance, K., & Byers, S. (1995). Sexual satisfaction in long-term heterosexual relationships: The interpersonal exchange model of sexual satisfaction. *Personal Relationships, 2*(4), 267–85.

Levine, M., & Troiden, R. (1988). The myth of sexual compulsivity. *Journal of Sex Research, 25*, 347–63.

Mayers, K. S., Heller, B. A., Heller, J. A. (2003). Damaged sexual self-esteem: A kind of disability. *Sexuality and Disability, 21*(4), 269–82.

Robinson, B. E., Bockting, W. O., Rosser, B. R., Miner, M., & Coleman, E. (2002). The sexual health model: Application of a sexological approach to HIV prevention. *Health Education Research, 17*(1), 43–57.

Rosser, B. R. S., Dwyer, S. M., Coleman, E., Miner, M., Metz, M., Robinson, B. E., & Bockting, W. O. (1995). Using sexually explicit material in sex education: An eighteen year comparative analysis. *Journal of Sex Education and Therapy, 21*, 117–28.

Runtz, M. (2003). *Child sexual abuse and sexual revictimization in young women*. Retrieved September 21, 2005, from http://web.uvic.ca/psyc/runtz/istssposter.ppt.

Sears, J. (1992). *Sexuality and the curriculum: The politics and practices of sexuality education*. New York: Teachers College Press.

Sexuality Information and Education Council of the United States. (1990). Position statements. *SIECUS Report, 4*(4), 10–12.

Shapiro, B. & Schwarz, J. (1997). Date rape: Its relationship to trauma symptoms and sexual self-esteem. *Journal of Interpersonal Violence, 12*(3), 407–19.

Stayton, W. R. (1998). A curriculum for training professionals in human sexuality using the sexual attitude restructuring (SAR) model. *Journal of Sex Education and Therapy, 23*, 26–32.

Stevenson, M. (1996). Sexual addiction: Disease or denigration? *Journal of Sex Research, 33*(2), 166–68.

Van Bruggen, L., Runtz, M., & Kadlec, H. (2006). Sexual revictimization: The role of sexual self-esteem and dysfunctional sexual behaviors. *Child Maltreatment, 11*(2), 131–45.

Wiederman, M., & Hurst, S. (1998). Body size, physical attractiveness, and body image among young adult women: Relationships to sexual experience and sexual esteem. *Journal of Sex Research, 35*(3), 272–81.

Wollert, R. (1978). A survey of sexual attitude reassessment and restructuring seminars. *Journal of Sex Research, 14*(4), 250–59.

World Health Organization. (1975). *Education and treatment in human sexuality: The training of health professionals*. WHO Technical Report Series 572. Geneva: World Health Organization.

Young, M., Luquis, R., Denny, G., & Young, T. (1998). Correlates of sexual satisfaction in marriage. *Canadian Journal of Human Sexuality, 7*, 115–28.

Zeanah, P., & Schwartz, J. (1996). Reliability and validity of the Sexual Self-Esteem Inventory for Women. *Psychological Assessment, 3*(1), 1–15.

CHAPTER 2

Braun-Harvey, D. (2009). *Sexual health in drug and alcohol treatment: A group facilitators manual*. New York: Springer.

Braun-Harvey, D. (2010). *Sexual health in recovery: A professional counselor's manual*. New York: Springer.

Bruess, C., & Greenberg, J. (2004). *Sexuality education: Theory and practice*. Boston: Jones & Bartlett.

Canadian Federation for Sexual Health. (2011). *How to talk about sex with your clients*. Retrieved September 1, 2011, from http://www.cfsh.ca/Your_Sexual_Health/How_to_Talk_about_Sex/With_Clients.

Center for Health Training. (2011). *Sexual history taking*. Retrieved September 1, 2011, from http://www.centerforhealthtraining.org/calendar/onlinetrainings/vid_sht/vid_sht.html.

Institute of Behavioral Research, Texas Christian University. (2011). *Manuals*. Retrieved September 1, 2011, from http://www.ibr.tcu.edu/pubs/trtmanual/manuals.html.

James, R. (2011). Correlates of sexual self-esteem in a sample of substance abusing women. *Journal of Psychoactive Drugs, 43*(3), 220–28.

Najavits, L. (2002). *Seeking safety: A treatment manual for PTSD and substance abuse*. New York: Guilford Press.

Silberman, M. (2006). *Active training: a handbook of techniques, designs, case examples, and tips*. San Francisco, CA: Jossey-Bass/Pfeiffer.

CHAPTER 3

Anderson, S. (2009). *Substance use disorders in lesbian, gay, bisexual, and transgender clients: Assessment and treatment*. New York: Columbia University Press.

Asay, T. P., & Lambert, M. J. (1999). The empirical case for the common factors in therapy: Quantitative findings. In M. A. Hubble & B. L. Duncan (Eds.), *The heart and soul of change: What works in therapy* (pp. 23–55). Washington, DC: American Psychological Association.

Cass, V. (1979). Homosexual identity formation: A theoretical model. *Journal of Homosexuality, 4*, 219–35.

Cass, V. (1984). Homosexual identity formation: Testing a theoretical model. *Journal of Sex Research, 20*(2), 143–67.

Center for Substance Abuse Treatments. (2001). *A provider's introduction to substance abuse treatment for lesbian, gay, bisexual and transgender individuals*. Rockville, MD: U.S. Department of Health and Human Services.

Cox, S., & Gallois, C. (1996). Gay and lesbian identity development: A social identity. *Journal of Homosexuality 30*(4), 1–30.

DiPlacido, J. (1998). Minority stress among lesbians, gay men, and bisexuals: A consequence of heterosexism, homophobia and stigmatization. In G. M. Herek (Ed.), *Stigma and sexual orientation: Understanding prejudice against lesbians, gays and bisexuals* (pp. 138–59). Thousand Oaks, CA: Sage.

Eliason, M. J. (2000). Substance abuse counselor's attitudes regarding lesbian, gay, bisexual, and transgendered clients. *Journal of Substance Abuse, 12*(4), 311–28.

Grossman, A. H. (1997). Growing up with a "spoiled identity": Lesbian, gay and bisexual youth at risk. *Journal of Gay and Lesbian Social Services, 6*, 45–60.

Hellman, R. E., & Drescher, J. (2004). *The handbook of LGBT issues in community mental health.* Binghamton, NY: Haworth Medical Press.

Hughes, T., & Wilsnack, S. (1997). Use of alcohol among lesbians: Research and clinical implications. *American Journal of Orthopsychiatry, 67*(1), 20–36.

Kinsey Institute. (2011). *Data from Alfred Kinsey's studies.* Retrieved September 1, 2011, from http://www.kinseyinstitute.org/research/ak-data.html#Findings.

Levine, H. (1997). A further exploration of the lesbian identity development process and its measurement. *Journal of Homosexuality, 34*(2), 67–78.

Lewis, C., Saghir, M., & Robins, E. (1982). Drinking patterns in homosexuality and heterosexual women. *Journal of Clinical Psychiatry, 43*, 277–79.

McKirnan, D. J., & Peterson, P. L. (1989). Alcohol and drug use among homosexual men and women: Epidemiology and population characteristics. *Addictive Behaviors, 14*, 545–53.

Michael, R., Gagnon, J., Laumann, E., & Kolata, G. (1994). *Sex in America: A definitive survey.* New York: Little, Brown.

Morales, E., & Graves, M. (1983). *Substance abuse: Patterns and barriers to treatment for gay men and lesbians in San Francisco.* San Francisco: San Francisco Prevention Resource Center.

Riddle, D. (1985). "Homophobia scale." Unpublished.

Skinner, W. (1994). Prevalence and demographic predictors of illicit and licit drug use among lesbians and gay men. *American Journal of Public Health, 84*, 1307–10.

Skinner, W., & Otis, M. (1996). Drug and alcohol use among lesbian and gay people in a southern U.S. sample: Epidemiological, comparative and methodological finding from the Trilogy Project. *Journal of Homosexuality, 30*(3), 59–62.

Sophie, J. (1986). A critical examination of stage theories of lesbian identity development. *Journal of Homosexuality, 12*(2), 39–51.

Wampold, B. E. (2001). *The great psychotherapy debate: Models, methods and findings.* Hillsdale, NJ: Lawrence Erlbaum Associates.

CHAPTER 4

Bandura, A. (1977). Self-efficacy: Toward unifying a theory of behavioral change. *Psychological Review, 84*(2), 191–215.

Bandura, A. (1982). Self-efficacy: Mechanism in human agency. *American Psychologist, 37*(2), 122–47.

Bartholomew, N. G., Rowan-Szal, G., Chatham, L. C., & Simpson, D. D. (1994). Effectiveness of a specialized intervention for women in a methadone program. *Journal of Psychoactive Drugs, 26*, 249–55.

Braun-Harvey, D. (2009). *Sexual health in drug and alcohol treatment: A group facilitators manual.* New York: Springer.

Camp, J. M., & Finklestein, N. (1997). Parenting training for women in residential substance abuse treatment: Results of a demonstration project. *Journal of Substance Abuse Treatment, 14*, 411–22.

Gomberg, E. (1994). Risk factors for drinking over a woman's lifespan. *Alcohol Health and Research World, 18*(3) 220–26.

Masters, W. H., & Johnson, V. E. (1966). *Human sexual response.* Boston: Little, Brown.

Mumme, D. (1991). Aftercare: Its role in primary and secondary recovery of women from alcohol and other drug dependence. *International Journal of the Addictions, 26*, 549–64.

Norwinski, J. (1993). *Hungry hearts: On men, intimacy, self-esteem, and addiction.* New York: Lexington Books.

Prochaska, J., DiClemente, C., & Norcross, J. (1992). In search of how people change: Applications to addictive behaviors. *American Psychologist, 47*(9), 1002–14.

Volpe, J., & Hamilton, G. (1982–1983). How women recover: Experience and research observations. *Alcohol Health and Research World, 7*(2), 28–39.

Wincze, J. P., & Carey, M. P. (2001). *Sexual dysfunction: A guide for assessment and treatment.* New York: Guilford Press.

CHAPTER 5

American Social Health Association. (2005). *Overview fact sheet on sexually transmitted diseases.* Retrieved November 20, 2005, from http://www.ashastd.org.

Centers for Disease Control. (2004). *HIV/AIDS surveillance report.* Retrieved December 28, 2004, from http://www.cdc.gov/hiv/stats/hasr1302/commentary.htm.

Centers for Disease Control (2009a). *2009 Sexually transmitted diseases surveillance, gonorrhea.* Retrieved July 14, 2011, from http://www.cdc.gov/std/stats09/gonorrhea.htm.

Centers for Disease Control (2009b). *2009 sexually transmitted diseases surveillance, syphilis.* Retrieved July 14, 2011, from http://www.cdc.gov/std/stats09/syphilis.htm.

Centers for Disease Control (2009c). *Trends in sexually transmitted diseases in the United States: 2009 national data for chlamydia, gonorrhea and syphilis.* Retrieved July 14, 2011, from http://www.cdc.gov/std/stats09/trends.htm.

Erikson, K., & Trocki, K. (1994). Sex, alcohol and sexually transmitted diseases: A national survey. *Family Planning Perspectives, 26*(6), 257–63.

Feroli, K., & Burstein, G. (2003). Adolescent sexually transmitted diseases. *American Journal of Maternal Child/Nursing, 28*, 113–18.

Gilgun, J., & Gordon, S. (1983). The role of values in sex education programs. *Journal of Research and Development in Education, 16*, 27–33.

Hayes, R., & Schultz, R. (1992). *What proportion of HIV infections are attributable to genital ulcers in sub-Sahara Africa?* Paper presented at the Eighth International Conference on AIDS, Amsterdam.

Hitchcock, J. (1996, March 27). The witch within me. *Newsweek*, 16.

Johnson, B., Carey, M., Marsh, K., Levin, K., & Scott-Sheldon, L. (2003). Interventions to reduce sexual risk for human immunodeficiency virus in adolescents, 1985–2000. *Archives of Pediatric and Adolescent Medicine, 157*, 381–88.

Mortens, T., Hayes, R., & Smith, P. (1990). Epidemiological methods to study the interaction between HIV infection and other sexually transmitted diseases. *AIDS, 4*, 57–65.

Pepin, J., Plummer, F., Brunham, B., Piot, P., Cameron, D., & Ronalds, A. (1989). The interaction of HIV infection and other sexually transmitted diseases: An opportunity for intervention. *AIDS, 3*, 3–9.

Prochaska, P., DiClemente, C., & Norcross, J. (1992). In search of how people change: Applications to addictive behaviors. *American Psychologist, 47*(9), 1102–14.

Seal, D. (1997). Interpartner concordance of self-reported behavior among college dating couples. *Journal of Sex Research, 34*, 39–55.

Tao, G., Irvine, K., & Kassler, W. (2000). Missed opportunities to assess sexually transmitted diseases in U.S. adults during routine medical check-ups. *American Journal of Preventive Medicine, 18*, 109–14.

Wasserheir, J. (1991). Epidemiological synergy: Interrelationships between HIV infection and other STDs. In L. Chen (Ed.), *AIDS and women reproductive health* (pp. 47–72). New York: Plenum Press.

CHAPTER 6

Bass, E., & Davis, L. (1994). *The courage to heal: A guide for women survivors of child sexual abuse* (new updated 3rd ed.). New York: HarperCollins.

Berliner, L., & Elliot, D. (1996). Sexual abuse of children. In J. Briere, L. Berliner, J. A. Buckley, C. Jenny, & T. Reids (Eds.), *The APSAC handbook on child maltreatment* (pp. 51–71). Thousand Oaks, CA: Sage.

Braun-Harvey, D. (1997). Sexual dependence among recovering substance-abusing men. In S. L. A. Straussner & E. Zelvin (Eds.), *Gender and addictions: Men and women in treatment* (pp. 359–84). New York: Rowman & Littlefield.

Browne, A., & Finkelhor, D. (1986). Impact of child sexual abuse: A review of the research. *Psychology Bulletin, 99*, 66–67.

Bryer, J., Nelson, B., Miller, J., & Krol, P. (1987). Childhood sexual and physical abuse as factors in adult psychiatric illness. *American Journal of Psychiatry, 144*, 1426–30.

Carnes, P., & O'Hara, S. (2000). *The Women's Sexual Addiction Screening Test (W-SAST)*. Retrieved October 16, 2011, from http://www.sexualrecovery.com/sri_docs/wsast.htm.

Cyder, M. A., Flory, K., Rainer, S., & Smith, G. T. (2009). The role of personality dispositions to risky behavior in predicting first-year college drinking. *Addiction, 104*, 193–202.

Eisenman, R., Dantzker, M. L., & Ellis, L. (2004). Self-ratings of dependency/addiction regarding drugs, sex, love and food: Male and female college students. *Sexual Addiction and Compulsivity, 11*, 115–27.

Finkelhor, D. (1979). *Sexually victimized children*. New York: The Free Press.

Finkelhor, D., & Browne, A. (1985). The traumatic impact of child sexual abuse: A conceptualization. *American Journal of Orthopsychiatry, 55*, 530–41.

Finkelhor, D., Hotaling, O., Lewis, I., & Smith, C. (1990). Sexual abuse in a national survey of adult men and women: Prevalence, characteristics, and risk factors. *Child Abuse and Neglect, 14*, 19–28.

Grice, D., Brady, K., Dustan, L., Malcom, R., & Kilpatrick, D. (1995). Sexual and physical assault history and post-traumatic stress disorder in substance-dependent individuals. *American Journal of Addictions, 4*, 297–305.

Hack, T. F., Osachuk, T. A. G., & DeLuca, R. V. (1994). Group treatment for sexually abused preadolescent boys. *Families in Society, 75*(4), 217–28.

Hansen, D. J., Hecht, D. B., & Futa, K. T. (1998). Child sexual abuse. In V. B. Van Hasselt & M. Hersen (Eds.), *Handbook of psychological treatment protocols for children and adolescents* (pp. 153–78). Mahwah, NJ: Lawrence Erlbaum Associates.

Heffernan, K., & Cloitre, M. (2000). A comparison of posttraumatic stress disorder with and without borderline personality disorder among women with a history of child sexual abuse: Etiological and clinical characteristics. *Journal of Nervous and Mental Disease, 188*, 589–95.

Irons, R., & Schneider, J. P. (1996). Differential diagnosis of addictive sexual disorders using the DSM-IV. *Sexual Addiction and Compulsivity, 3*, 7–21.

Irvine, J. (1995). Reinventing perversion: Sex addiction and cultural anxieties. *Journal of the History of Sexuality, 5*, 429–40.

Kendall-Tackett, K. A., Williams, L. M., & Finkelhor, D. (1993). Impact of sexual abuse on children: A review and synthesis of recent empirical studies. *Psychological Bulletin, 113*(1), 164–80.

Klein, M. (2002). Sex addiction: A dangerous clinical concept. *Electronic Journal of Human Sexuality, 5* (n.p.).

Levine, M., & Troiden, R. (1988). The myth of sexual compulsivity. *Journal of Sex Research, 25*, 347–63.

Lewis, M. (1992). *Shame: The exposed self.* New York: Free Press.

Neddermeyer, D. (2011). *Sexual abuse myths.* Retrieved October 16, 2011, from http://drdorothy.info/?page_id=54.

Norris, J., Stoner, S. S., Hessler, D. M., Zawacki, T., Davis, K. C., George, W. H., et al. (2009). Influences of sexual sensation seeking, alcohol consumption, and sexual arousal on women's behavioral intentions related to having unprotected sex. *Psychology and Addictive Behavior, 23*, 14–22.

Parker, B., & McFarlane, J. (1991). Nursing assessment of the battered pregnant woman. *American Journal of Maternal Child Nursing, 16*, 161.

Perera, B., Reece, M., Monahan, P., Billingham, R., & Finn, P. (2009). Relations between substance use and personal dispositions towards out-of-control sexual behaviors among young adults. *International Journal of Sexual Health, 21*, 87–95.

Reinhart, M. A. (1987). Sexually abused boys. *Child Abuse and Neglect, 11*, 229–35.

Rind, B., & Tromovitch, P. (1997). A meta-analytic review of findings from national samples of psychological correlates of child sexual abuse. *Journal of Sex Research, 34*, 237–55.

Schmidt, C. (1999). Sex and addiction: Are there addictive features to sex behavior? *Medical Crossfire Debate.* Available: http://www.medicalcrossfire.com/debate_archive/1999.

Scott, W. (1992). Group therapy with sexually abused boys: Notes toward managing behavior. *Clinical Social Work Journal, 20*(4), 395–409.

Seegers, J. A. (2003). The prevalence of sexual addiction symptoms on the college campus. *Sexual Addiction and Compulsivity, 10*, 247–58.

Sirles, E. A., Walsma, J., Lytle-Barnaby, R., & Lander, L. C. (1988). Group therapy techniques for work with child sexual abuse victims. In *Violence: Prevention and treatment in groups* (pp. 67–78). New York: Haworth.

Spacarrelli, S. (1994). Stress, appraisal, and coping in child sexual abuse: A theoretical and empirical review. *Psychological Bulletin, 116*, 340–62.

Spelman, C. (1993). *Talking about childhood sexual abuse.* Chicago: National Committee to Prevent Child Abuse.

Swett, C., Surrey, J., & Cohen, C. (1990). Sexual and physical abuse histories and psychiatric symptoms among male psychiatric outpatients. *American Journal of Psychiatry, 147*, 632–36.

Vanderbilt, H. (1992, February). *Incest: A chilling report.* New York: LEAR Publishing.

Wilsnack, S., Vogeltanz, N., Klassen, A., & Harris, T. (1997). Childhood sexual abuse and women's substance abuse: National survey findings. *Journal of Studies on Alcohol, 58*, 264–71.

Windle, M., Windle, R., Schedit, D., & Miller, G. (1995). Physical and sexual abuse and associated mental disorders among alcoholic inpatients. *American Journal of Psychiatry, 152*, 1322–28.

Women's Web. (2011). *Child sexual abuse/incest.* Retrieved September 13, 2011, from http://www.womensweb.ca/violence/incest/effects.php.

Zamanian, K., & Adams, C. (1997). Group psychotherapy with sexually abused boys: Dynamics and interventions. *International Journal of Group Psychotherapy, 47*(1), 109–26.

CHAPTER 7

Boles, S. M., & Johnson, P. B. (1997). Gender, weight concerns, and adolescent smoking. *Journal of Addictive Disorders, 20*(2), 5–14.

Cash, T. F., Ancis, J. R., & Strachan, M. D. (1997). Gender attitudes, feminist identity, and body images among college women. *Sex Roles, 37*, 433–47.

Croll, J. (2007). *Body image and adolescents: Guidelines for adolescent nutritional services.* Retrieved June 21, 2011, from http://www.epi.umn.edu/let/pubs/img/adol_ch13.pdf.

Croll J., Neumark-Sztainer D., Story, M., & Ireland M. (2002). Prevalence and risk and protective factors related to disordered eating behaviors among adolescents: Relationship to gender and ethnicity. *Journal of Adolescent Health, 31*, 166–75.

Forman, M., & Davis, W. N. (2005). Characteristics of middle-aged women in inpatient treatment for eating disorders. *Eating Disorders, 13*, 231–43.

French, S. A., Perry, C. L., Leon, G. R., & Fulkerson, J. A. (1994). Weight concerns, dieting behavior, and smoking initiation among adolescents: A prospective study. *American Journal of Public Health, 84*(11), 1818–20.

Granner, M. L., & Black, D. R. (2001). Racial differences in eating disorder attitudes, cigarette and alcohol use. *American Journal of Health Behavior, 25*(2), 83–99.

Kearney-Cooke, A. (2002). Familial influences on body image development. In T. F. Cash & T. Pruzinsky (Eds.), *Body image: A handbook of theory, research, and clinical practice* (pp. 99–107). New York: Guilford Press.

Kinnier, R. T., Metha, A. T., Okey, J. L., & Keim, J. (1994). Adolescent substance use and psychological health. *Journal of Alcohol and Drug, 40*(1), 51–56.

Krahn, D., Piper, D., King, M., Olson, L., Kurth, C., & Moberg, C. P. (1996). Dieting in sixth grade predicts alcohol use in ninth grade. *Journal of Substance Abuse, 8*(3), 293–301.

Leit, R. A., Pope, H. G., & Gray, J. J. (2001). Cultural expectations of muscularity in men: The evolution of Playgirl centerfolds. *International Journal of Eating Disorders, 29*(1), 90–93.

Natenshon, A. (2006). *Early warning signs of eating disorders in classrooms, corridors, lunch rooms and guidance offices.* Retrieved June 22, 2011, from: http://www.empoweredparents.com/1school eatingdisorders/school_01.htm.

Natenshon, A. (2011). *Recognizing early warning signs of disease.* Retrieved June 22, 2011, from: http://www.abigailnatenshon.com/ recognizing.aspx.

National Association of Social Workers. (2001). Adolescent girls and body image. *Adolescent Health, 2*(4). Retrieved June 22, 2011 from: http://socialworkers.org/practice/adolescent_health/ah0204.asp.

National Eating Disorders Association. (2005). *National Eating Disorders Association statistics: Eating disorders and their precursors.* Retrieved June 20, 2011, from http://www.nationaleatingdisorders .org/uploads/file/Statistics%20%20Updated%20Feb%2010, %202008%20B.pdf.

National Institute on Aging. (2006). *Dramatic changes in U.S. aging high-lighted in new census, NIH report: Impact of baby boomers antici-pated.* Retrieved June 20, 2011, from http://www.nia.nih.gov/NewsAndEvents/PressReleases/PR2006030965PlusReport.htm.

Nieri, Z. T., Kulis, S., Keith, V. M., & Hurdle, D. (2005). Body image, acculturation, and substance abuse among boys and girls in the south-west. *American Journal of Drug and Alcohol Abuse, 31*(4), 617–39.

Peat, C., Peyerl, N., & Muehlenkamp, J. (2008). Body image and eating disorders in older adults: A review. *Journal of General Psychology, 135*(4), 343–58.

Poncelet, B. (2009). *Mom, am I fat? Helping your teen have a positive body-image.* Retrieved June 22, 2011, from http://www.Teen%20Body%20Image%2020Encouraging%20Positive%20Teen%20Body%20Image.webarchive.

Rand, C. S. W., & Wright, B. A. (2000). Continuity and change in the evaluation of ideal and acceptable body sizes across a wide age span. *International Journal of Eating Disorders, 28*, 90–100.

Raudenbush, B., & Zellner, D. A. (1997). Nobody's satisfied: Effects of abnormal eating behaviors and actual and perceived weight status on body image in males and females. *Journal of Clinical Psychol-ogy, 16*, 95–110.

Scheier, L. M., Botvin, G. J., Griffin, K. W., & Diaz, T. (2000). Dynamic growth models of self-esteem and adolescent alcohol use. *Journal of Early Adolescence, 20*(2), 178–209.

Siegel, J. M. (2002). Body image change and adolescent depressive symp-toms. *Journal of Adolescent Research, 17*(1), 27–41.

U.S. Department of Health and Human Services. (2009). *Body image and your kids: Your body image plays a role in theirs.* Retrieved June 10, 2011, from http:/www.womanshealth.gov.

Wilcox, S. (1997). Age and gender in relation to body attitudes. *Psychol-ogy of Women Quarterly, 21*, 549–65.

Wilson, T. G. (1999). Eating disorders and addiction. *Drugs and Society, 15(1/2)*, 87–102.

CHAPTER 8

American Psychiatric Association. (1994). *Diagnostic and statistical manual of mental disorders* (4th ed.). Washington, DC: Author.

Beck, J. G. (1995). Hypoactive sexual desire disorder: An overview. *Jour-nal of Consulting and Clinical Psychology, 63*, 919–27.

Beckman, L. (1979). Reported effects of alcohol on the sexual feelings and behavior of women alcoholics and non-alcoholics. *Journal of Studies on Alcohol, 40*, 272–82.

Blume, S. (1991). Sexuality and stigma: The alcoholic woman. *Alcohol Health and Research World, 15*, 139–46.

Bullough, V. L. (1976). *Sexual variance in society and history*. Chicago: University of Chicago Press.

Bullough, V. L. (2001). Masturbation as a means of achieving sexual health. In W. O. Bockting & E. Coleman (Eds.), *Masturbation as a means of achieving sexual health* (pp. 17–33). New York: Haworth Press.

Cado, S., & Leitenberg, H. (1990). Guilt reactions to sexual fantasies during intercourse. *Archives of Sexual Behavior, 19*, 49–63.

Cass, V. (1979). Homosexual identity formation: A theoretical model. *Journal of Homosexuality, 4*, 219–35.

Coleman, E. (2002). Masturbation as a means of achieving sexual health. In W. O. Bockting & E. Coleman (Eds.), *Masturbation as a means of achieving sexual health* (pp. 5–16). New York: Haworth Press.

Covington, S., & Kohen, J. (1984). Women, alcohol and sexuality. *Advances in Alcohol and Substance Abuse, 4*(1), 41–56.

Donahey, K. M., & Carroll, R. A. (1993). Gender differences in factors associated with hypoactive sexual desire. *Journal of Sex and Marital Therapy, 19*, 25–40.

Fink (Eds.) *Contemporary marriage: Special issues in couples therapy* (pp. 241–260). Homewood, IL: Dorsey.

Hurlbert, D. F. & Whittaker, K. A. (1991). The role of masturbation in marital and sexual satisfaction: A comparative study of female masturbators and nonmasturbators. *Journal of Sex Education & Therapy, 17*(4), 272–82.

Kaplan, H. S. (1975). *The illustrated manual of sex therapy*. New York: Brunner/Mazel.

Kelly, R. J., & Freysinger, V. J. (2000). *21st century leisure: Current issues*. Boston: Allyn & Bacon.

Kontula, O., & Haavio-Mannila, E. (2002). Masturbation in a generational perspective. In W. O. Bockting & E. Coleman (Eds.), *Masturbation as a means of achieving sexual health* (pp. 49–83). New York: Haworth Press.

Peugh, J., & Belenko, S. (2001). Alcohol, drugs and sexual function: A review. *Journal of Psychoactive Drugs, 33*(3), 223–32.

Schaefer, S., & Evans, S. (1987). Women, sexuality and the process of recovery. In E. Coleman (Ed.), *Chemical dependency and intimacy dysfunction* (pp. 91–120). New York: Haworth Press.

Singer, J. L. (1966). *Daydreaming*. New York: Random House.

Stayton, W. R. (1985). Alternative lifestyles: Marital options. In D. C. Goldberg & P. J. Finks (Eds.), *Contemporary marriage: Special issues in couples therapy* (pp. 241–60). Homewood, IL: Dorsey.

Wilsnack, S. (1991). Sexuality and women's drinking. *Alcohol, Health and Research World, 15*(2), 147–50.

World Association of Sexology. (1999). *Declaration of sexual rights*. Retrieved September 10, 2011, from http://www.sexology.it/declaration_sexual_rights.html.

CHAPTER 9

Bagley, C., & Tremblay, P. (1997). Suicidal behaviors in homosexual and bisexual males. *Crisis, 19*(1), 24–34.

Booth, A., Johnson, D. R., & Granger, D. A. (1999). Testosterone and men's health. *Journal of Behavioral Medicine, 22*(1), 1–19.

Charnetski, C. C., & Brennan, F. X. (2001). *Feeling good is good for you: How pleasure can boost your immune system and lengthen your life*. Emmaus, PA: Rodale Press.

Clayton, A. H., & Cantor-Cooke, R. (2007). *Satisfaction: Women, sex, and the quest for intimacy*. New York: Ballantine.

Coleman, E. (2002). Masturbation as a means of achieving sexual health. *Journal of Psychology and Human Sexuality, 14*(2/3), 5–16.

Covington, S. (1991). Sororities of helping and healing: Women and mutual self-help groups. In P. Roth (Ed.), *Alcohol and other drugs are women's issues* (pp. 85–92). Metuchen, NJ: Scarecrow Press.

Covington, S. (2002). Helping women recover: Creating gender-responsive treatment. In S. Straussner & S. Brown (Eds.), *The handbook of addiction treatment for women: Theory and practice* (pp. 52–72). San Francisco: Jossey-Bass.

Cutler, W. B. (1991). *Love cycles: The science of intimacy*. New York: Villard Books.

Davey Smith, G., Frankel, S., & Yarnell, J. (1997). Sex and death: Are they related? Findings from the Caerphilly cohort study. *British Medical Journal, 315*(7123), 1641–44.

Ebrahim, S., May, M., McCarron, P., Frankel, S., & Davey, S. (2002). Sexual intercourse and risk of ischaemic stroke and coronary heart disease: The Caerphilly study. *Journal of Epidemiology and Community Health, 56*(2), 99–102.

Ellison, C. R. (2000). *Women's sexualities*. Oakland, CA: New Harbinger Publications.

Fogari, R., Zoppi, A., Preti, P., Rinaldi, A., Marasi, G., Vanasia, A., & Mugellini, A. (2002). Sexual activity and plasma testosterone levels in hypertensive males. *American Journal of Hypertension, 15*(3), 217–21.

Gaynor, P. & Underwood, J. (1995). Conceptualizing and measuring sexual self-esteem. In Shrout, P., Fiske, S., *Personality research, methods and theory: a festcrift honoring Donald W. Fiske*. NJ: Hillsdale.

Harrison, D., & Pennel, C. (1989). Contemporary sex roles for adolescents: New options or confusion? *Journal of Social Work and Human Sexuality, 8*, 27–46.

James, R. (2011). Correlates of sexual self-esteem in a sample of substance abusing women. *Journal of Psychoactive Drugs, 43*(3), 220–28.

Jorgensen, S. (1983). Beyond adolescent pregnancy research frontiers for early adolescent sexuality. *Journal of Early Adolescence, 3*, 141–55.

Komisaruk, B. R., & Whipple, B. (1995). The suppression of pain by genital stimulation in females. *Annual Review of Sex Research*, 151–86.

Laumann, E. O., Gagnon, J. H., Michael, R. T., & Michaels, S. (1994). *The social organization of sexuality: Sexual practices in the United States*. Chicago: University of Chicago Press.

Lê, M. G., Bacheloti, A., & Hill, C. (1989). Characteristics of reproductive life and risk of breast cancer in a case control study of young nulliparous women. *Journal of Clinical Epidemiology, 42*(12), 1227–33.

Levin, R. J. (2002). The physiology of sexual arousal in the human female: A recreational and procreational synthesis. *Archives of Sexual Behavior, 31*(5), 405–11.

Meaddough, E. L., Olive, D. L., Gallup, P., Perlin, M., & Kliman, H. J. (2002). Sexual activity, orgasm and tampon use are associated with a decreased risk for endometriosis. *Gynecologic and Obstetric Investigation, 53*, 163–69.

Miller, J. B. (1986). *What do we mean by relationships?* (Work in Progress No. 22). Wellesley, MA: Stone Center.

Ogden, G. (2001). Spiritual passion and compassion in late-life sexual relationships. *Electronic Journal of Human Sexuality*. Retrieved September 15, 2011, from: http://www.ejhs.org/volume4/Ogden.htm.

Palmore, E. (1982). Predictors of the longevity difference: A twenty-five year follow-up. *The Gerontologist, 22*, 513–18.

Persson, G. (1981). Five-year mortality in a 70-year old urban population in relation to psychiatric diagnosis, personality, sexuality and early parental death. *Acta Psychiatrica Scandinavica, 64*, 244–53.

Petridou, E., Giokas, G., Mucci, L. A., & Trichopoulos, D. (2000). Endo-
crine correlates of male breast cancer risk a case control study in
Athens, Greece. *British Journal of Cancer, 83*(9), 1234–37.

Planned Parenthood Federation of America, Inc. (2003). *White paper: The
health benefits of sexual expression*. Published in cooperation with
the Society for the Scientific Study of Sexuality. New York: Kather-
ine Dexter McCormick Library.

Richmond-Abbot, M. (1983). *Masculine and feminine roles over the life
cycle*. Reading, MA: Addison-Wesley.

Robinson, B., Bockting, W., Rosser, B. R., Miner, M., & Coleman, E.
(2002). The sexual health model: Application of a sexological
approach to HIV prevention. *Health Education Research, 17*(1),
43–57.

Sayle, A. E., Savitz, D. D., Thorp, J., Hertz-Picciotto, I., Wilcox, A. J., &
Allen, J. (2001). Sexual activity during late pregnancy and risk of
preterm delivery. *Obstetrics and Gynecology, 97*(2), 283–89.

Schaffer, K. (1981). *Sex roles and human behavior*. Cambridge, MA:
Withrop.

Seal, A. Minichiello, V., & Omodeo, M. (1997). Young women's sexual
risk taking behavior: Re-visiting the influences of sexual self-
efficacy and sexual self-esteem. *International Journal of STD &
AIDS, 8*(3), 159–65.

Shapiro, B. & Schwarz, J. (1997). Date rape: Its relationship to trauma
symptoms and sexual self-esteem. *Journal of Interpersonal
Violence, 12*(3), 407–19.

Snell, W., & Papini, D. (1989). The sexuality scale: An instrument to measure sexual self-esteem, sexual depression, and sexual preoccupation. *Journal of Sex Research, 26*, 256–63.

Weeks, D. J. (2002). Sex for the mature adult: Health, self-esteem and
countering ageist stereotypes. *Sexual and Relationship Therapy,
17*(3), 231–40.

Weeks, D., & James, J. (1998). *Secrets of the superyoung*. New York:
Berkley Books.

Wilsnack, S. (1991). Sexuality and women's drinking. *Alcohol, Health
and Research World, 15*(2), 147–50.

Winter, L. (1988). The role of sexual self-concept in the use of contracep-
tives. *Family Planning Perspectives, 20*(3), 123–27.

Zamboni, B. D., & Crawford, I. (2002). Using masturbation in sex
therapy: Relationships between masturbation, sexual desire, and sexual fantasy. *Journal of Psychology and Human Sexuality, 14*(2/3),
123–41.

Zeanah, P., & Schwartz, J. (1996). Reliability and validity of the sexual self-esteem inventory for women. *Psychological Assessment, 3*(1), 1–15.

CHAPTER 10

Advocates for Youth. (2011). *The circles of human sexuality*. Retrieved September 1, 2011, from http://www.advocatesforyouth.org/for-professionals/lesson-plans-professionals/198?task=view.

Brown, L., & Gilligan, C. (1992). *Meeting at the crossroads: Women's psychology and girls' development*. New York: Ballantine Books.

Chodorow, N. (1999). *The reproduction of mothering: Psychoanalysis and the sociology of gender*. Berkeley: University of California Press.

Gilligan, C. (1993). *In a different voice: Psychological theory and women's development*. Cambridge, MA: Harvard University Press.

Kostova, E. (2010). *The swan thieves*. New York: Little, Brown & Co.

Mahler, M., Pine, F., & Bergman, A. (2000). *The psychological birth of the human infant*. New York: Basic Books.

Meltzer, B. (2011). *The inner circle*. New York: Grand Central Publishing.

Miller, J. B. (1976). *Toward a new psychology of women*. Boston: Beacon Press.

Miller, J. B. (1991). The development of women's sense of self. In J. V. Jordan, A. G. Kaplan, J. B. Miller, I. P. Stiver, & J. L. Surrey (Eds.), *Women's growth in connection: Writings from the Stone Center* (pp. 11–26). New York: Guilford Press.

O'Neil, J. (2006). Helping Jack heal his emotional wounds: The gender role conflict diagnostic schema. In M. Englar-Carlson & M. S. Stevens (Eds.), *In the room with men: A casebook of therapeutic change* (pp. 259–84). Washington, DC: American Psychological Association.

Pollack, W. S. (1995). No man is an island: Toward a new psychoanalytic psychology of men. In R. F. Levant & W. S. Pollack (Eds.), *A new psychology of men* (pp. 33–67). New York: Basic Books.

Schilit, R., & Gomberg, E. (1987, Summer). Social supports structures of women in treatment for alcoholism. *Health and Social Work, 12* (3), 187–95.

Surrey, J. (1991). Relationship and empowerment. In J. V. Jordan, A. G. Kaplan, J. B. Miller, I. P. Stiver, & J. L. Surrey (Eds.), *Women's growth in connection: Writings from the Stone Center*. New York: Guilford Press.

Yalom, I. D. (1970). *The theory and practice of group psychotherapy*. New York: Basic Books.

CHAPTER 11

Braun-Harvey, D. (2009). *Sexual health in drug and alcohol treatment: A group facilitators manual.* New York: Springer.

Gilgun, J., & Gordon, S. (1983). The role of values in sex education programs. *Journal of Research and Development in Education, 16,* 27–33.

Hill, P. C., Pargament, R. W., MCCullough, M. E., Swyers, J. P., Larson, D. B., & Zinnbauer, B. J. (2000). Conceptualizing religion and spirituality: Points of commonality, points of departure. *Journal for the Theory of Social Behaviour, 30*(1), 51–77.

Runtz, M. (2003). *Child sexual abuse and sexual revictimization in young women.* Retrieved September 21, 2005, from http://web.uvic.ca/psyc/runtz/istssposter.ppt.

Shapiro, B., & Schwarz, J. (1997). Date rape: Its relationship to trauma symptoms and sexual self-esteem. *Journal of Interpersonal Violence, 12*(3), 407–19.

Wulff, D. M. (1991). *Psychology of religion.* New York: Wiley.

CHAPTER 12

Bird, J. & Bird, L. (1976). *Sexual loving.* New Jersey: Doubleday.

Braun-Harvey, D. (2009). *Sexual health in drug and alcohol treatment: A group facilitator's manual.* New York: Springer.

Braun-Harvey, D. (2010). *Sexual health in recovery: A professional counselor's manual.* New York: Springer.

Index

About the Author

Raven L. James, PhD, is a sexologist, researcher, professor, and author and has worked professionally in the field of addiction and sexual health since 1994. She has conducted research on sexual self-esteem in the addiction treatment process, behavioral therapies development, sexual abuse, sexual orientation, gender, and more. She has published numerous peer-reviewed journal articles, a book chapter, and developed training curricula, including HIV Prevention, Human Sexuality, Dying and Death, STD Counseling Issues, and Working with LGBT Issues in Substance Abuse Treatment.

Dr. James currently teaches at Governors State University near Chicago, Illinois, in a Master of Health Science in Addictions Studies Program, where she participates in community-based research, regularly presenting her research at statewide and national conferences. She holds active membership in several professional organizations, including the International Coalition for Addiction Studies Education, the International Association of Relationship Research, and the Society for the Scientific Study of Sexuality.

Raven was a master trainer and prevention professional for the New York State Office of Alcohol and Substance Abuse Services. Her community-based work in New York State included assistant director of education for an AIDS organization and peer coordinator for a substance abuse prevention agency.

James believes that "our sexuality is a sacred part of who we are as human beings. We need to embrace our individuality and honor our stories in order to be healthy and happy."